The Posthuman Condition

The Posthuman Condition

Ethics, Aesthetics and Politics
of Biotechnological Challenges

Edited by
Kasper Lippert-Rasmussen, Mads Rosendahl Thomsen
and Jacob Wamberg

AARHUS UNIVERSITY PRESS

The Posthuman Condition
MatchPoints 3
© the authors and Aarhus University Press
Typeset by Narayana Press
Cover by Jørgen Sparre (after Lisbet Tarp's illustration)
    Image from Colourbox.com
Printed by Narayana Press, Denmark
Printed in Denmark 2012
ISBN 978 87 7934 570 6
ISSN 1904-3384

Aarhus University Press

Aarhus
Langelandsgade 177
DK – 8200 Aarhus N

Copenhagen
Tuborgvej 164
DK – 2400 Copenhagen
www.unipress.dk

Published with the financial support of
The Aarhus University Research Foundation

INTERNATIONAL DISTRIBUTORS:

Gazelle Book Services Ltd.
White Cross Mills
Hightown, Lancaster, LA1 4XS
United Kingdom
www.gazellebookservices.co.uk

ISD
70 Enterprise Drive
Bristol, CT 06010
USA
www.isdistribution.com

Contents

■ Posthuman Horizons and Realities: Introduction

Kasper Lippert-Rasmussen, Mads Rosendahl Thomsen and Jacob Wamberg

Even though Homo sapiens during the last century and a half have, by and large, come to terms with being the result of a long and amazing evolution, until recently there has not been much speculation about the future prospects of humanity as we know it. The pace of Charles Darwin's evolution by natural selection is very slow and what the successors to this most-advanced species may turn out to be has been too speculative a question to really matter. However, in the past two decades, this perspective has shifted as a number of astounding technological developments have taken place. These developments have the power to completely overturn human evolution from its dependency on unplanned mutations and natural selection to an artificial evolution where conscious decisions and technological design matter more – thus setting the direction for an array of minor and major changes in both the human as well as other species. This shift promises a profound transformation of humanity and society as a whole, indeed of the entire life of our planet, and thus it has received a quite dramatic name: the posthuman.

The interdisciplinary field emerging around the idea of the posthuman had a less radical forerunner in posthumanism, a movement already imploding the anthropocentric perspective of the humanities since the 1960s: either negatively as an anti-humanistic deconstruction of the idea of the human subject, or positively as an ecological orientation focusing on life in all its varieties (Badmington 2011: 374). The posthuman thus signifies a move from posthumanism's agenda, which was purely conceptual, to a mixed field of theory and practice where interventions of biotechnology supposedly will change the human species to something clearly separate from the human being we know. An intermediate step towards such a development is often referred to as "transhuman" which signifies individuals that bear strong non-human traits, as for example cyborgs or chimeras (Savulescu 2010: 214). Although this notion concerns a passage in which the prosthetic enhancements of the body have not yet dissolved the idea of the human subject altogether, the transhuman is to an even greater degree than the posthuman permeated by utopian expectations.

Prior to 1990 the term "posthuman" was rarely used, and even though science fiction and futuristic philosophies of technology have conjured up numerous visions of new humans, the idea of a radical change in life conditions and essential traits of the species did not set a broader agenda. In the past decade and a half, however, it has become a thriving subject where very different approaches and visions intersect and where science and medicine as well as philosophy, law, art, literature and psychology all contribute with unique perspectives. It is a field that deals with both imminent uses of new technologies and more long-term conjectures about the human species. In both cases it produces scenarios that test the limits of what is commonly considered ethical.

The posthuman essentially revolves around the key ethical dilemmas made acute by technological advances. In spite of recurrent doubts in many parts of societal debates as to whether technology actually improves civilization or not – from the ancient myths of civilization's technologically conditioned decadence to Theodor W. Adorno, Maurice Merleau-Ponty and Martin Heidegger's pessimistic notions of rationalistic technology colonizing the life world – it is a widely held belief in parliamentary politics, 'third world' development strategies and large parts of popular culture that most of the options technology facilitates are beneficial: that longer lives, better health, and accelerated actions are desirable. This confidence in technological progress is a significant heritage of the Enlightenment thinking, and in many ways it runs smoothly together with other aspects of the optimistic view of humankind's progressive evolution.

However, turning to the inherent rights for every human being expressed in the UN's Universal Declaration of Human Rights (1948), the question is how progression towards a *posthuman* universalism can coexist with the idea of every human's value as expressed in the declaration. Are individuals with an even higher dignity possible? Or is it so that human dignity is corrupted by biotechnological enhancement of the human body? In a recurrent reference in this book, *Our Posthuman Future* from 2002, Francis Fukuyama has no doubts. Drawing upon dystopian visions such as those put forward in Aldous Huxley's *Brave New World* (1932), Fukuyama insists that certain core values of the human subject are so complex and irreducible to simple dogmas that a biotechnological attempt to alter their foundations could lead to disastrous results (Fukuyama 2002: 218).

It seems reasonable to not only relate Fukuyama's worries to a distant future, but to keep the issue in mind even today. A number of biotechnologies have already presented us with a range of bewildering ethical questions, and promise to do so even more comprehensively in the future. The most important are the following developments: *The advanced diagnosis of genes*, which will affect which foetuses will be allowed to grow and enter the world as humans. Some selections will be seen as generally permissible, whereas others will be seen as a step towards intolerance and dehumanizing. *Advances in medicine* will likely create the possibility of better health and longer lives, but could also lead to shortages of access to treatments and a risk of an even greater divide within societies and between the more and less developed countries. *General longevity* will rise, and this process will increase the proportion of elderly people in society significantly and provoke questions of life quality in old age: What is a human life and is longer necessarily better? Another important development is the ability to make *spare body parts*. This already greatly advanced field is one in which necessary concerns will most likely query the limits of our (known) authentic human subject. Likewise, the *interaction between humans and machines,* increasingly seen in e.g. the treatment of deafness and the enhancement of disabled people's motor skills, could, when and if used by people with no disabilities, dissolve the borders between the autonomous human and its surroundings. Questions of *genetic engineering* now taking place on a small scale could quickly expand and spark dizzying ethical implications with for example three would-be parents use in an attempt to eliminate the risks of inherited diseases. In many other instances the therapeutic ends of this procedure are generally considered justified, whereas attempts to make enhancements are viewed sceptically. As a final development we see how the possibility of *cloning* humans technically is within reach. This is obviously closely connected to a whole host of challenges of technical risks – as well as questions of moral respect for humankind as a species.

It is, indeed, fair to guess that many other techniques and dilemmas, now barely imaginable, are waiting in our horizon. Although the idea of a human essence in a Platonic sense has largely been given up philosophically, all these techniques ironically bring something like this essence to the fore again. However, its contours are not easily seen. Rather, the human constitutes a hazy shell confronted with imperatives of using technology to strengthen the human species *and* warnings about doing so.

The limits of knowledge and key conflicts

Advances in technology are the driving force behind the agenda of bioethics and the posthuman horizon, but the numerous uses and side-effects are so far-reaching that they affect almost every discipline – and with questions that can be answered from very different angles: Can beauty be part of a moral argument concerning choices one wants to make for oneself as well as for others? Is societal cohesion a valid reason for restricting the freedom of the individual? Would societies with huge differences in life expectancy be acceptable? How much of a 'cyborg' would we allow an individual human being to become? Nature clones – but can we? And of course, who are the "we" that should decide? The pervasive nature of such questions, coupled with the uncertainty of future developments, means that this field comprises a number of different research domains.

Immanuel Kant's tri-part division of questions into "What can we know? What ought we to do? For what may we hope?" is informative in order to show the complexities of the subject (Kant 1974: 677). First of all, what can we know? There are many predictions that involve huge uncertainties, from the effects of certain technologies to the way human identity and societal development will play out. The great variation in the precision of previous predictions of the future suggests that making projections about the future based on present conditions is a very risky thing to do. On the other hand, there are so many technologies that are already being implemented and so many experiments being carried out on animals and humans that a whole array of developments could be predicted based on those with which we are already familiar. Also, we have already seen a number of somewhat bizarre constellations of human-technology enhancements, which now may seem superfluous but which in a futuristc perspective greatly expand the possible field of evolutionary diversity and selection.

Obviously, Kant's question of what is (ethically and morally) right to do is in many ways the most complex to answer. The dilemmas presented above are echoed in the schism between technophilia and technophobia: whether human evolution and progress is something that should be striven for with all means at hand, or whether the complexity is too dense to even initiate. Perhaps it would be better to leave the matter out of human hands, but, as implied in the outline above, this argument is essentially untenable and irrelevant today, where the complexities of the uses of technology cannot rightfully be reduced to a matter of total inclusion or exclusion. A number of enhancing technologies already exists today, and the either/or reduction is not a choice: enhancements are a matter of degree. Today the general approach to the implementation of new technology is cautiousness with a strong focus on therapy rather than enhancement. But is this middle way between rejection or even reluctance and embracement the right way to proceed – also from a moral standpoint?

Finally, as new possibilities arise, the focus of Kant's question of what we may hope for changes. Often the answers gravitate towards what *not* to hope for, as portrayed in many dystopian novels, films and in other arts. Again, this is a field where the difference between the grand visions of a very different future can seem unattached to small steps towards better living conditions, but when examined more closely, the accumulation of many small steps could end up with a situation not hoped for. Hence the difficulties in articulating a valuable political stance that encompasses the many conflicts – while knowing that a strong political stance is indeed necessary.

In this volume the approaches taken to the many dilemmas and conflicts of the posthuman condition range from probing technical possibilities and artistic visions to examining ethical problems and exploring political considerations. Four conflicts are in focus throughout. Divided between analytical and ethical concerns, these conflicts include (1) the gradual nature of changes, (2) the kinds of changes that are possible, and at what speed they arrive, (3) individual freedom and societal cohesion, and (4) human nature and future identities.

(1) Technology changes the conditions of human existence in various dimensions. Some changes may not produce anything that would be considered posthuman, since the technologies involved are embodied but do not become fully integrated parts of the body. Similarly, the engineering in question, for instance in genetics, takes place on a small scale with no perceptible immediate consequences for our everyday experience.

Even if the link between artificial and natural is still not strong enough (or the scale is not large enough) to seriously make us question whether someone is a cyborg or a human, such uses are part of a shift from a qualitative idea of human anatomies as strictly natural to a *sliding scale of change*, in which technologically modified human bodies may constitute something beyond the human. If genetically engineered or modified individuals were to become the norm, even for the purpose of avoiding inherited diseases, would that signify a break with humanity as we know it? Would enhanced humans be humans if they were to acquire significant other features such as a double lifespan, almost perfect memory and a vastly improved intelligence?

(2) What changes are possible – ranging from minor but perhaps not wholly innocent changes such as improved eyesight, to radical changes of the human DNA or the *de facto* migration of humans into non-biological life, as futurist Ray Kurzweil envisions in *The Singularity is Near: When Humans Transcend Biology* from 2005? The question is intricately bound up with a temporal dimension, a horizon of expectation: When do the posthuman techniques actually take over? Both the short-term and the long-term scenarios are important here, as they both influence policy making.

In the temporal perspective one could distinguish between two kinds of technological scepticists. One scepticist, the pragmatic, would argue that technology does not keep its promises and that the cloning of people, the uploading of entire brains or "merely" cures for deadly diseases are not as imminent as one could be led to believe, but that they would be welcome. Thus, even if promises are not kept, the path towards partial gains should still be followed. Another scepticist, the full-grown one represented by Francis Fukuyama among others, would on the contrary celebrate such broken promises because this scepticist does not believe technological opportunities can bring advances for humankind, given the complexity of human existence.

(3) Entering more explicitly into the ethical dilemmas, one conflict is between

individual freedom and societal cohesion. Many scenarios of human evolution consider the possibility of the co-existence of humans and posthumans. Imagine the above-mentioned society with differing aging possibilities – say, where some people live four or five times longer than the majority – and how that would affect ethics.

A more immediate impact of conflict between individual freedom and societal considerations lies in the use of prenatal analysis, which is bound to become more complex and wide-ranging. Two cases illustrate how this affects societies today. In societies where boys are generally valued more than girls, there have been astonishing and unnatural discrepancies in birth rates between the sexes: no less than sixty percent more male births than female births have been reported in parts of China. This creates significant issues not least for adult men who cannot find female partners, while rising crime rates also have been reported.

The effects of such interventions are not limited to what doctors do to foetuses, but transmit to how entire societies cope with new situations created by widespread use of technology. If extensive genetics analysis and selection were to become widespread, it could very well alter general perceptions of what is natural and what is valuable. However, it is also possible to imagine that tolerance would grow even if the band of the normal becomes narrower.

(4) Finally, the question of human nature and the future identities of humans is ubiquitous in the debate. Many posthuman technologies involve benefits as well as risks, and while it should not be forgotten that this is true of existing technologies as well (e.g. burning coal has benefits but also risks such as irreversible and harmful global warming), the intrusion into the very bodily existence of humans makes a difference to most people. Art and literature have long provided numerous examples of scenarios that imagine alternative visions for humans, just as artists themselves have invested their bodies in experiments with new technologies. Even if the idea of human identity has been challenged, it is still at the centre of many reflections on values and universalism. The posthuman horizon only attracts more attention to the grounds on which human identity is founded or constructed.

Humans are complex beings who cannot easily break away from what their genes have allowed them to become – although their cultural software may be very adaptable. But the new sense of a greater control or promises of control have set a new agenda for considering what human nature is, if it even makes sense to talk of a "nature". In any case, there will be visions of selfhood and identity that will be nurtured and evolved, but in which direction? No one – neither the natural scientist nor the humanist nor the layman – has the answer.

The articles in this volume

This book is divided into four sections. "Technological scenarios" deals with both the near future and long term visions of changes. "Ethical dilemmas" addresses different cases that highlight the complexities of making clear-cut decisions of what is right and wrong. "Artistic responses" provides three examples of how art and literature contribute to the envisioning, and perhaps even practice, of the future of humanity. Finally, "Political responses" delivers three conflicting arguments on how societies should react towards the technological possibilities.

(1) Technological scenarios

As described above, the question of the posthuman is entangled with a number of different technologies that either already influence our world or may well do so in a near future. There is a great leap from improved medicine to the creation of cyborgs or genetical modification, but there is also a continuum in which the uses of the available technologies are just as important.

Chris Hables Gray opens the volume by addressing the interactions between man and machine which produce hybrid beings known as cyborgs. Gray's view is that it is essentially human not to be at home in our bodies, thereby adopting a point of departure which is very different from the typical assumption that machines are alien to the natural body. Evoking a long view on human existence, he suggests that we see man's integration with technology as a consequence of the social foundation for the rapid evolutions of mankind's capabilities in the past 10,000 years. A more evolved awareness of what Gray terms "cyborg citizenship" is thus a precondition for an inclusive and reflected use of the technologies that are continually being put into use in human existence.

This generalized view of the cyborg stands in striking contrast to the escatological expectations found in many places in the current debate on transhumanism. As demonstrated in Maxwell Mehlman's contribution, the question of immortality is central to the hopes of transforming humans through genetic engineering. In the transhumanist rhetoric of a never ending life in good health Mehlman identifies an ironic quasi-religious element that is hard to distinguish from traditional narratives of Paradise. Yet Mehlman shows how risky and uncertain the tampering with genes is and is likely to remain, as the sources of fatal errors are numerous.

Lone Frank describes a series of effects that our increasing knowledge of genetics is having and is likely to have in the future. Her starting point is the relatively low cost of gene sequencing, which enables people to seek out information about their own DNA and the risks that they may carry with them. This increased knowledge may lead to new viewpoints of what it means to be human, some more reductive than one might hope for. Nevertheless, it is likely that knowledge of how genes determine or strongly influence what we become will lead to different perspectives on identity. She also considers how attitudes towards diversity will evolve: diversity is heralded as a positive concept, but discrimination and even racism are also part of human history. Frank's conclusion is that increased knowledge of one's own genetics will be another aspect of the existential search for identity and a tool for better understanding of what we do with our bodies and codes.

Finally, while stressing the fallibility of predicting the future, Søren Holm provides an overview of likely scenarios for the advances of medicine in a relatively near future (the next 25 years), and in a somewhat more distant future a century away. He stresses that the future will be marked by an array of different technologies and warns against simplifying the situation by focusing on a single technology that will make all the difference. Longevity will rise significantly although by no means create sensations of immortality, and there will still be diseases that cannot be cured. However, medicine will be much more effective and will take advantage of our knowledge of genes and ability to create personalized medicine. Holm also predicts that enhancement will be common with respect to sensory, motor and cognitive functions. But while the gradual lowering of the cost of initial treatments will make them accessible to more people, medicine of the future will not reach all those who need it.

(2) Ethical dilemmas

The issue of posthumanity is widely believed to raise a large number of important ethical dilemmas, i.e. cases of technological possibilities which may both be ethically defended and attacked and whose outcome is utterly undetermined. Indeed, in many cases it might not even be clear which reasons favour or disfavour realizing what has become technologically feasible. Some might think that discussions of ethical dilemmas in relation to the use of new technologies are irrelevant in the sense that if some people would benefit from the introduction of these technologies they will be used, wherever the balance of moral reasons lies. However, this is not always the case. Some people would prefer to engage in human cloning, and yet for ethical reasons it is banned in almost all countries. Also, the EU has, in effect, banned GMOs. Non-ethical interests do not *wholly* determine which technologies are used.

Three contributions to this book address posthuman ethical dilemmas. First, Sarah Chan and John Harris locate the prospect of posthumanity and the ways in which posthumans might come into being in a broader setting. They caution that ethical issues raised by this prospect are much less significant than many think. Indeed, they conjecture that a gradual transition from humanity to posthumanity will happen largely unnoticed and is in any case to be embraced. It should, however, encourage us to rethink our present moral attitudes towards species boundaries and towards other biological species. One worry is that we inflate the moral significance of belonging to the human species and that, given a suitably uninflated view, many of the ways in which we treat animals, e.g. in industrialized agriculture, are morally indefensible.

Second, Kasper Lippert-Rasmussen considers genetic "enhancements" that benefit their targets by making sure that they do not have features (for instance a particular sexuality, gender or disability) that result in them suffering discrimination at the hands of others. In one view, to "enhance" human beings in these dimensions would be to treat symptoms of unjust social norms. What we should do instead is to address the underlying causes of the norm, i.e. the existence of prejudiced social rules pertaining to disabilities etc., by reconfiguring these norms. This may not always be feasible, however, and Lippert-Rasmussen argues that it is morally permissible for individual couples to use discrimination-dependent genetic enhancements of their future child even though the state should often forbid individual couples from exercising this moral permissibility (in which case it may become impermissible for individual couples to use enhancement techniques, not because doing so is wrong in itself but because, ex hypothesis, doing so is illegal).

Third, Lene Bomann-Larsen takes issue with permissive liberal views which claim that the state should not prevent parents from designing, modifying or selecting genes for the purpose of improving the traits and endowments of their children, provided that such actions do not harm others in morally problematic ways. She defends a more restrictive liberal view where the state may restrict parental freedom, because the state must respect the claim of children as future citizens – political persons with entitlements – and these rights include not just a right not to be harmed, but also a right to be treated as sovereign individuals who are entitled to an open future. The latter right implies that enhancement *may* wrong future citizens even when carried out in order to *benefit* them – and even when it does actually benefit them.

(3) Artistic responses
Our models of the future development of technology and its interventions in culture are very much dependent on fiction and art. In artistic representations and presentations, known and yet unknown meetings between body and artefacts can be extrapolated and unfolded in those complicated knots of ethical, social, scientific and existential dimensions, which easily escape our attention in the more specialized domains of science and even philosophy.

In his article, Mads Rosendahl Thomsen draws on the theory of autopoetics systems by sociologist Niklas Luhmann. His theory discerns between three kinds of systems that use the distinction between themselves and their environment as part of their way of operating: biological organisms, psychic systems and social systems. From this division Thomsen follows the idea of a new human in literature, arguing that the new human had three dominant phases in the 20th century. From the ambitions post-Nietzschean hopes of changing spiritual life and perceiving the world in different ways, to the historically devastating attempts of refining the exiting humans through a change of societies, to the posthuman horizon that focuses on bodily changes. Writers such as Virginia Woolf, Mo Yan and Don DeLillo have all explored how fragile ideas of human identity gain complexity and relevance through the exploration of life-story narratives that must present a concrete relation to cultural history and ideas of selfhood.

In Gert Balling's contribution the lens is turned to visual art, as well as more explicitly to the transformed human body in a perspective of information technology. Analyzing two cases of digitally manipulated photographs – Nancy Burson's average human types, from beauty ideals to dictators, and Keith Cottingham's fictitious portraits of perfect male youths – Balling invokes a new function for art, one moving from a metaphorical to an implementable level. In the performances of the Australian artist Stelarc, future scenarios of machines meeting flesh are in fact explored in a remarkably physical manner; although Balling also remarks on a certain retro quality linking the performances with sci-fi classic such as Fritz Lang's *Metropolis*. The body is transformed, opened and linked to internet movements through heavy cables and robotic prosthetics, stressing the alien quality of a technology to which we easily become too accustomed.

However, the question of art's relation to the posthuman is not merely a question of mirroring future scenarios – it also involves intervening in them. As Jacob Wamberg shows in his contribution, the principles of artistic creation could in fact themselves prove to be crucial in the future evolution of both technology and nature. Setting off from two neo-Hegelian scenarios of the end of history – Francis Fukuyama's political protection of the human subject against posthuman intervention and Arthur C. Danto's art-philosophical protection of the autonomous artwork against mere thingness – Wamberg dynamizes the Hegelian teleology by transforming it into a posthuman passage, in which consciousness and its cultural products meet and are interlaced with their former other: natural evolution. Drawing upon the continental philosophies of Schelling, Schopenhauer and Bergson, Wamberg considers that this meeting practically activates those unconscious forces of nature which in modernity before 1900 could enter cultural artefacts only in the abstracted form of artistic representations, but which in the last century have entered the environment through the interactive experiments of avant-garde art.

(4) Political possibilities
How should society regulate the use of various technologies for the improvement of human capacities, e.g. cognitive enhancements? Francis Fukuyama thinks many such uses should be forbidden. He stresses how the complexity of humans that

have evolved as a species through thousands of years entails significant risks of unintended results should germ-line engineering become more widespread. Another reason for adopting a cautious approach to enhancement is that it might challenge the cohesion of societies. Societies might become more unequal, leading to an unintended threat to their overall function. In the light of this, he delivers an argument against the idea that regulation is futile and that technologies will be used once they exist. Drawing upon historical examples such as the international limitation of nuclear arms and the existence of regulatory systems within medicine, Fukuyama is quietly optimistic about the possibility of maintaining a democratic control of the uses of biotechnology, which in the end may have the result that there will not be a posthuman future.

In his contribution Torbjörn Tännsjö defends normative egalitarianism about cognitive capacities. According to this view, we should not seek to boost human cognitive capacities *per se*, but should reduce the variation in the cognitive capacities of human beings by levelling up to a point within the normal human range the cognitive capacities of those who fall below the normal human range, e.g. those with an IQ below 80. Tännsjö argues that this position can be defended on a number of different grounds. From a utilitarian point of view Tännsjö's proposal is likely to reduce the gap between what people have the capacity to do and what they want to do, thereby reducing frustration and boosting happiness. However, Tännsjö also argues that this view is consistent with Fukuyama's right-based approach that focuses on human dignity, despite the fact that Fukuyama apparently suggests the contrary. Specifically, given the modest egalitarianism of Tännsjö's scheme, it does not involve the creation of a hierarchical society of enhanced super-humans and ordinary human beings. Indeed, it will rather eliminate the present situation in which some human beings have much lower cognitive capacities than others.

Like Torbjörn Tännsjö, Julian Savulescu addresses the way in which technologies can be used to serve egalitarian purposes. Acknowledging that equality will never be achieved in any society, he argues that our present society is already so complex that large groups of people find the performance of common tasks such as filling in their tax returns to be so difficult that they are deprived of having "a fair go" at achieving a good life. In this light, Savulescu addresses the means of cognitive enhancements and the possibility that they could give more people the ability to cope with the demands of society. At the same time, it should not be ruled out that the enhancement of humankind's moral basis and relationships with people outside the closest circles is an area for improvement that may also be technologically possible. Well aware that there may not be an absolute limit to when enhancement is enough, Savulescu also touches upon what he calls "radical possibilities" in which genetic engineering could provide completely new physical capabilities.

Exit?

The question of the posthuman is at once urgent and speculative. On the one hand, it deals with questions that are imminent and changes that are going on right now, unobtrusively establishing new standards of what is normal and what is not. On the other, it makes an inquiry into what the general direction of human existence should be in the light of our current opportunities to advance the conditions of the human race – while risking tampering with the near-universally held dignity of human existence. But what if the path to achieving dignity goes through the embracement of technological advances?

This volume does not even intend to lead to firm conclusions, but seeks to highlight the diversity of positions that exist and to point to how they link certainty and uncertainty about uses of technology, conflicting notions of human values and societal justice as well as emotions of whether this field represents a trauma or an enchantment.

Even though evolutionary theory gives us every reason to believe that humans will only exist for a limited time in the history of the Earth – and that it would be the natural course to arrive at something well beyond the human – the posthuman condition is perhaps not given as something that will necessarily happen through biotechnological means. Nevertheless, the posthuman is a horizon that has been established more firmly than ever before in the history of humankind. It is a horizon that may remain a horizon for a long time, but it may also be a horizon that will disappear with the arrival of a posthuman condition.

References

Badmington, Neil (2010) "Posthumanism", in B. Clarke and M. Rossini (eds) *The Routledge Companion to Literature and Science*, London: Routledge.

Fukuyama, Francis (2002) *Our Posthuman Future: Consequences fo the Biotechnological Revolution*. New York: Farrar, Straus and Giroux.

Huxley, Aldous (1932) *Brave New World*, London: Chatto and Windus.

Kant, Immanuel (1974) *Kritik der reinen Vernunft*, Suhrkamp: Frankfurt am Main.

Savulescu, Julian (2010) "The Human Prejudice and the Moral Status of Enhanced Beings: What Do We Owe the Gods?", in J. Savulescu and N. Bostrom (eds) *Human Enhancement*, Oxford: Oxford University Press.

"Universal Declaration of Human Rights", http://www.un.org/events/humanrights/2007/hrphotos/declaration%20_eng.pdf.

Notes on contributors

Gert Balling is a special adviser at the Danish Ministry of Science, Innovation and Higher Education. He did his PhD at the IT University in Copenhagen. He has been involved in a number of anthologies and articles on technology transfer and technology in broader contexts and has won several awards for science mediation.

Sarah Chan is Deputy Director of ISEI (Institute for Science, Ethics and Innovation) and Research Fellow in Bioethics and Law at the University of Manchester. She has published widely on human enhancement and bioethics.

Lene Bomann-Larsen did her PhD and post.doc at the University of Oslo, where her last project was on challenges from the sciences to conceptions of freedom and moral responsibility. She has published on this topic in Neuroethics and Criminal Law and Philosophy, as well as in several anthologies. She is currently Associate Professor and Research Coordinator at the Norwegian Military Academy. Her main research interest lies in the ethics of war, and she is an associate editor of the *Journal of Peace Research*.

Lone Frank is a journalist and author with a PhD in neurobiology and a background in research. She has written for leading international publications such as Science, Nature Biotechnology and Newsweek and regularly appears as a commentator on Danish radio and television. She is the author of four books: *The New Life*, *Cloned Tigers*, *Mindfield*, and *My Beautiful Genome*.

Francis Fukuyama is Olivier Nomellini Senior Fellow at the Freeman Spogli Institute for International Studies, Stanford University. He was a member of the US Bioethics Council from 2001-2004, and is the author of *Our Posthuman Future: Consequences of the Biotechnology Revolution*. His most recent book is *The Origins of Political Order: From Prehuman Times to the French Revolution*.

Chris Hables Gray is Professor of Graduate Studies for The Union Institute and University and lectures at UCSC. His research focuses on pragmatic and cultural studies of information, especially in terms of war, peace, cyborgs and evolution. He publishes in journals such as *Cultural Politics*, *Teknokultura*, and *Science as Culture*. Currently he is finishing his latest book, entitled *Infoisms: Aphorisms on Information*, and beginning his next, *Taking Evolution Seriously*.

John Harris FMedSci, is Director of The Institute for Science, Ethics and Innovation and of the Wellcome Strategic Programme in The Human Body, its Scope Limits and Future, University of Manchester, where is he is Lord Alliance Professor of Bioethics. Books Include: *Clones Genes and Immortality*. 1998. John Harris (ed.). 2001. *Bioethics*. Oxford Readings in Philosophy Series. Justine C. Burley and John Harris (eds.). 2002. *A Companion To Genethics: Philosophy and the Genetic Revolution*. (Blackwell's Companions to Philosophy series). *On Cloning*. 2004. *Enhancing Evolution* was published by Princeton University Press in 2007.

Søren Holm is Professor of Bioethics at the University of Manchester, where he directs the Centre for Social Ethics and Policy. He also holds a part-time Chair in Medical Ethics at the Centre for Medical Ethics, University of Oslo. He works primarily in bioethics and the philosophy of medicine. He is the current Editor-in-Chief of *Clinical Ethics.*

Maxwell J. Mehlman is the Arthur E. Petersilge Professor of Law and Director of the Law-Medicine Center at Case Western Reserve University School of Law, and Professor of Bioethics at Case Western Reserve University School of Medicine. His new book, *Transhumanist Dreams and Dystopian Nightmares: Genetic Engineering and the Future of Human Evolution*, will be published in the fall of 2012 by Johns Hopkins University Press.

Kasper Lippert-Rasmussen is Professor of Political Theory at Aarhus University. He works primarily in political and moral philosophy and has published in journals such as *Journal of Political Philosophy*, *Ethics*, *Philosophy and Public Affairs*, *Philosophical Studies*, *Economics and Philosophy*, and *The Journal of Ethics*. Presently he is working on a book-length manuscript on discrimination. He is an associate editor of *Ethics* and Chair of the Society for Applied Philosophy.

Julian Savulescu is Uehiro Chair in Practical Ethics at the University of Oxford. He directs the Oxford Uehiro Centre for Practical Ethics, the Oxford Centre for Neuroethics, and the Institute for Science and Ethics. He is Louis Matheson Distinguished Visiting Professor at Monash University, Honorary Professorial Fellow at the Florey Neuroscience Institutes and editor of the *Journal of Medical Ethics*. He is the author of over 170 publications in journals including *Bioethics, American Journal for Bioethics*, and *Journal of Applied Philosophy*. Presently he is working on a book for Oxford University Press with Ingmar Persson entitled *Unfit for the Future: The Need for Moral Enhancement.*

Torbjörn Tännsjö is Kristian Claëson Professor of Practical Philosophy at Stockholm University. He has published extensively in moral philosophy, political philosophy, and bioethics. Some of his published books are *Moral Realism, Conservatism for Our Time, Populist Democracy, Hedonistic Utilitarianism, Coercive Care, Understanding Ethics, Global Democracy*, and *From Reasons to Norms*.

Mads Rosendahl Thomsen is an Associate Professor in Comparative Literature at Aarhus University. He is the Director of the Danish Network for Cultural Memory studies and a member of Academia Europaea. He has published *Mapping World Literature: International Canonization and Transnational Literatures* and is a co-editor of *World Literature: A Routledge Reader*. He is finishing a book for Continuum entitled *The New Human in Literature: Visions of Changes in Body, Mind and Society after 1900*.

Jacob Wamberg is Professor of Art History at the Institute of Aesthetics and Communication at Aarhus University. He is currently working on post-1900 art in a perspective of biocultural evolution. His publications include *Landscape as World Picture: Tracing Cultural Evolution in Images, Art and Alchemy* (ed.) and *Totalitarian Art and Modernity* (co-edited with Mikkel Bolt Rasmussen).

PART I

TECHNOLOGICAL SCENARIOS

1 Cyborging the Posthuman: Participatory Evolution

> There can be little doubt that the fabrication of the cyborg is a sign of a collective anxiety around the ubiquitous presence of the machine. (Bruce Grenville 2001: 47)

> **i-cyborg:** 'We want to make Google the third half of your brain.' Co-founder Sergey Brin declared, while explaining the new search feature that guesses what the users want.
> (*San Francisco Chronicle*, Sept. 12 2010, E10)

Homo sapiens cyborg

If one accepts evolution, one must accept that humans will not last forever. *Homo sapiens sapiens* will one day be extinct, perhaps to be replaced by one or more posthuman species. While for most creatures evolution is driven by natural selection, there are a number of organisms, especially plants and animals, whose recent development has been determined by artificial selection exercised by humans. This includes us.

Humans evolved out of earlier primates over the last few million years. In the last 250,000 years this evolution has accelerated dramatically. There is growing evidence that environmental shifts have been crucial, especially about roughly 200,000 and 50,000 years ago and during the human expansion out of Africa since (Cochran and Harpending 2009).

What makes humans so different? Why are we so estranged from wild nature? We have no near neighbors on the tiny branch of the primates we occupy. *Homo erectus? Homo antecessor? Homo neanderthalensis?* Even *Homo sapiens idaltu?* Dead, dead and gone (Sarmiento 2007). Our distant cousins, chimps and bonobos, we can certainly feel affinity for, and some have become "companion species" (Haraway 2003) to humans. But the nature we truly love is what we have made: the dogs and cats, pink roses and fat red strawberries. These are all the result of our artificial selections. So is our culture, our human nature.

How our culture evolved is a matter of great debate. What role did the development of music play? Of language? (Anderson and Lightfoot 2002). What was crucial? The invention of war? (Wrangham and Peterson 1996; Ehrenrich 1997; Malcolm and Potts 2008). Of cooking? (Wrangham 2009). Fascinating as these debates are, the outlines of the incredible success of *Homo sapiens sapiens* is clear. Humans have used our invention and mastery of language, of tools (including fire), of companion animals and plants (agriculture), of tools to invent tools, of technology writ large (cities, armies), of writing, and of machines that can do things we cannot (fly, blow up whole cities, compute pi to a million places) to accelerate our evolution and dominate the world. The latest stage in this process, perhaps the final stage for humanity, is the integration of small artificial systems (vaccines, pacemakers, cochlear ear implants) into humans and of humans into larger technical systems.

This new relationship between our bodies, our minds, and our machines has been framed in a number of different ways. It has been called the vital machine (Channell 1991), the 4th Discontinuity (Mazlish 1993), radical evolution (Garreau 2005), and cyborg society (Gray 2001). The postmodern condition (Harvey 1990) is a more economic perspective and the hybrid is a common frame in science studies (Hard and Jamison 2005), so cyborgization is but one analytic. What makes it particularly useful is that it focuses on our evolving nature, and it contextualizes us as systems in systems, as weavers of systems. Unsurprisingly, it turns out the idea of the cyborg is central to contemporary psychology (Edwards 1996), economics (Mirowski 2002) and war (Gray 1997).

Humans are a protean animal, a modeling animal, the making and remaking animal, the naked ape (Morris 1980), the artificial ape (Taylor 2010), the civilized ("city living") ape, the augmented animal (Anderson 1996), clearly the cybernetic organic primate, the "natural-born cyborg" (Clark 2007). Humans are transforming the world from ecology to cybernetic organism, call it noosphere (Teilhard de Chardin 2004), metaman (Stock 1993), symbiont Gaia (Haraway 1995), global intelligence (Dyson 1998) or terminator singularity. Whatever you call it, it is an expression of what makes us. Cyborging is what humans do.

A cyborg is a cybernetic organism, which is any self-regulating (homeostatic) system that includes organic (living, natural, evolved) and machinic (unliving, artificial, invented) subsystems. The most important of these are modified humans, including, technically, anyone who has been vaccinated. But even the unvaccinated of the world, and there are not many, live in a human culture that is totally dependent on an incredible array of technosciences. We all live in a Cyborg Society mediated not just by profound human-machine integrations, but also by multiple mundane cyborgian relationships (Mentor 2010).

A cyborg can also be a biocomputer (with memory that can die), a transgenic plant (jellyfish genes in tomatoes, for instance), or a cockroach with electrodes in its head controlled by Japanese scientists.

Cyborgization is not limited to systems incorporating human elements, but

Figure 1. *Roboroach*, pencil sketch © Joshua Gray.
This real roach, modded by Japanese scientists with simple electrodes and electro-taught basic commands, is not a cyborg alone. It is part of a system of roach, machines, and human scientists that itself is a cyborg system. The drawing only shows part of the larger system, the experimental subject.

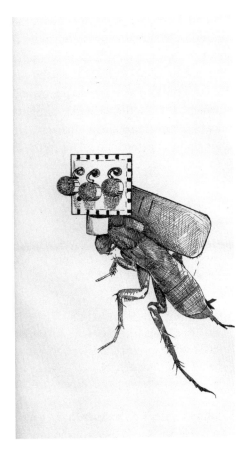

humans perform all cyborgizations and human-based cyborgs are the most interesting, whether it is the fantasy of Robocop, a maimed soldier with a sophisticated prosthetic arm, a dead person kept alive with machines awaiting organ harvesting (a neomort or living cadaver) or anyone whose immune system has been reprogrammed by vaccinations. There are many different types and levels of cyborgization. The incorporated living elements (viral, bacterial, plant, insect, reptile, rodent, avian, mammal), the technological interventions (vaccination, machine prosthesis, genetic engineering, nanobot infection, xenotransplant) and the level of integration (mini, mega, meta, mundane) can all vary, an infinite number of possible cyborgs, life multiplied by human invention and intervention. (Gray et al. 2010).

While millions use the internet, where every user is a temporary cyborg, and billions have been immunized, cyborgization is little known nor understood. Much of the most interesting theory is actually found in science fiction, but there is also a growing body of literature from critical and cultural studies, catalyzed by Donna Haraway's famous "Manifesto for Cyborgs" (1985). Her argument that cyborgization mandated a deeper engagement with the politics of technoscience and a challenge to simple dichotomous epistemologies has resonated broadly through many fields and disciplines. The politics of cyborgization is a subfield of its own, as in *Cyborg Citizen* (Gray 2001), *Our Posthuman Future* (Fukyama 2002) and *Citizen Cyborg* (Hughes 2004). There is also a growing literature about being cyborged, the best of which are from the wearable computer pioneer Steve Mann (2001) and the cochlear ear implant recipient Michael Chorost (2005). Their articulate and thoughtful adaptability is a good model for future *Homo sapiens cyborg*.

Shockwave Riders

... an uncanny experience occurs either when infantile complexes which have been repressed are once more revived by some impression, or when primitive beliefs which have been surmounted seem once more to be confirmed.

(Sigmund Freud 1919: 60)

When John Brunner first told me of his intention to write this book, I was fascinated – but I wondered whether he, or anyone, could bring it off. Bring it off he has – with cool brilliance. A hero with transient personalities, animals with souls, think tanks and survival communities fuse to form a future so plausibly alive it has twitched at me ever since.

(Alvin Toffler, Author of *Future Shock*, blurbing John Brunner's *Shockwave Rider* 1975)

In John Brunner's *Shockwave Rider*, a near-future dystopian world of disasters ruled by profiteers is saved by revolutionary computer hacking cyborgs so in tune to the quickly emerging world-wide "data-net" that they take it over and use it to bring a democratic form of e-government into being. Brunner was inspired, in part, by Alvin Toffler's *Future Shock* (1970), which argued that the pace of human change had become so great that the future, coming more quickly and forcefully upon us every day, was an autonomous power that had to be reckoned with, that it was a wave we had to learn to ride. Brunner's story is a decidedly radical take on what this means. In his bleak future, technoscientific revolution necessitates political revolution and that starts with taking evolution seriously.

We need to adapt to adapting since we live in the age of the institutionalization of innovation. We need to be shockwave riders because we are also shockwave makers. The number of scientists and engineers alive today is greater than all the scientists and engineers from the past. And today they have better technology, so inevitably the pace of technoscientific change is increasing geometrically.

This relentless, ubiquitous transformative future is producing a great dis-ease in our culture. As death has haunted humanity since sentience, so now does cyborgization permeate everything we think and do. Both call into question ourselves,

Figure 2. *Renaissance Cyborg,* ink drawing © Bob Thawley. *Homo sapiens cyborg* will be very familiar to most of us. Technically, they are a subspecies of *homo sapiens*, as we (*homo sapiens sapiens*) are. The same basic parameters will govern their existence: birth, survival, death, love. They may have mechanical prosthesis and complex vaccinations, maybe even a little genetic engineering, but they will be quite recognizable to Leonardo da Vinci's *The Vitruvian Man,* here upgraded by the San Francisco artist Bob Thawley.

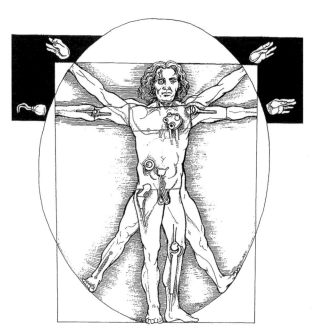

they make us look into the abyss, an uncanny valley. The uncanny valley is where creatures fall when they trigger recognition as human, but yet are not. Cyborgs join vampires, zombies, ghosts, androids and various shadows that go bump in the night in this disturbing zone (Diamond 2010). But cyborgs are real and they are us. This is profoundly disorienting. Similar disorienting major transformations of human consciousness/culture have occurred before: Taming Fire, Recognizing Death and Creating Story, Tools, Music, Language, Culture, Civilization and Machines were clearly on the same scale. Still, such ruptures are not common and this current break with the past could well herald the end of the human – in extinction or posthumanities. We feel the danger and the possibilities, the constant shock of the new, and behind wild dreams of immortality the inevitability of death.

So to be human is to feel uncanny. We are at home and not at home with our bodies. Because of the lens of consciousness, our very nature is familiar and yet uncomfortably strange. Our models of reality are always in tension with reality itself; a model cannot match reality, which is too complex to predict consistently anyway. Even that sliver of reality we have evolved to interact most with, the vulgar physics of the Newtonian model, of hunting and hunted at the water hole, is truly beyond our ken. Base desires, the blood and mucus and excrement of living, the inevitable totality of death, are concealed in our daily lives but always present. It is always there, the itch in our mind that cannot be soothed and now we see the future in our own faces in the mirror every morning.

In Brunner's book a few heroes save the world with one brilliant insight/intervention/invention. This meets the demands of Story, but it takes more than a few insights, or a few people, to shape the future. The possibilities of change are limited by our culture, of course, but also by the technical limits of cyborgization itself, the technoscientific processes that make it possible.

The real heroes of *Shockwave Rider* are the interlinked impossible technologies and deeply improbable networking skills that provide the appropriately deus ex machina happy ending. Real cyborgs are systems, and all systems of being and of knowing are profoundly limited. This is seen most clearly in formal systems. Kurt Gödel showed that the mother of all formal systems, mathematics, is limited because it is necessarily incomplete, or paradoxical, or both. The final option ("both") has not yet been proven – but it seems most likely. He did this by making a perfectly legitimate mathematical algorithm from the famous paradox of Greek philosophy about the Cretan liar. If a Cretan tells you he always lies then is that a lie? Ironically, the mathematics proves that the lie is that mathematics can be perfect. Alonzo Church and Alan Turing used the same trick to show that an infinite computer inevitably is incomplete, or has paradoxes, or both.

From physics we know that the observer always affects the system being observed: the Heisenberg Uncertainty Principle. And since the observer system is always changing (being observed itself, for example, when we ponder it), no system is static. An implication of this is the Bayesian Paradox: to know the position of an electron means one cannot know its path, or vice versa. In other words, we cannot know everything, and to know some things means not to know others.

Any non-trivial cyborg system is "out-of-control" in the sense that it cannot be controlled from outside, it has self-regulation, homeostasis. This is one of a number of insights from complexity theory on the unpredictable and uncontrollable aspects of complex systems, including all biological ones. Even if the artificial (machinic, genetic, nano) becomes a million times more complex and sophisticated, there will always be technological limits to the replacement of the biological by us. Gregory Bateson pointed out that a system cannot know itself. At best it can make a map, a model, but the map is never the territory. The tension between needing to believe in our stories, our models, our maps, and yet realize that *they are not reality* will never disappear. We need to embrace it, to ride it, for the repressed returns as irrationality or worse.

What is uncyborgable? By definition, parts of every cyborg have not been cyborged, that is the paradox at cyborg's heart. A cyborg is always biological, at least in some small way. When machines totally replace the biological, that will be a robot and the cyborg will be gone. But that is hard to imagine, the biologic is easily as adaptable as the machinic. As long as there are cyborgs, the organic will survive.

Fear, and desire, and other human emotions and choices will set limits on cyborgization, as will the very nature of systems and the realities of technology. But as an expression of human nature, our morphing, moding, messing around with our environment and ourselves, cyborgization is going to continue and deepen.

Cyborg Citizenship

A human child raised on a desert island with no social interaction would end up with the cognitive skills as an adult that are not very different from an ape's, because a lot of our really smart adaptations are adaptations for putting our heads together with others and learning from others.
(Michael Tomasello, Max Planck Institute for Evolutionary Anthropology, Flora 2010)

It is possible to evolve societies in which people live in greater freedom, exert greater influence on their circumstances, and experience greater dignity, self-esteem, purpose, and well being. The route to such a society must include struggles toward democratic institutions for evolving a more democratic technological order. Is it realistic to envision a democratic politics of technology? Isn't it unrealistic not too?
(Richard Sclove 1995: 244)

The issue isn't if we'll be cyborged, but how, and who will decide. As Donna Haraway proclaimed a quarter of a century ago – we must take responsibility for our cyborgorization (1985). We must take responsibility for our evolution. Otherwise, somebody else will. The Borg of the *Star Trek* universe is a good warning. If we don't chose participatory evolution, our future will not be guided by ourselves or even the blind hand of chance. Instead, tomorrow will be molded by the vulgar fist of governments, corporations and other authoritarian systems that in service of their short-term ends will warp us into nightmares. Here the Borg are wrong. Resistance isn't futile; resistance is fertile. Evolution is a series of revolutions (and vice versa); and now, if we participate consciously in our own evolution, we are the revolutionaries, like it or not.

New technologies mandate new political systems and institutions if democracy is to be preserved and deepened. Constitutions, Bills of Rights, and (self) governing initiatives are crucial democratic technologies, but so are autonomous decentralized organizations that cut across and below official systems to do directly what civil society or specific communities desire. These new political technologies are based only in part on old political theories. New theories, coming out of actual political struggles and practices and from artistic and technological innovations, are crucial. Theories about information, the sign/trope/hallmark of postmodernity, are particularly important.

The process that produces all cyborg technologies, including the political, fol-

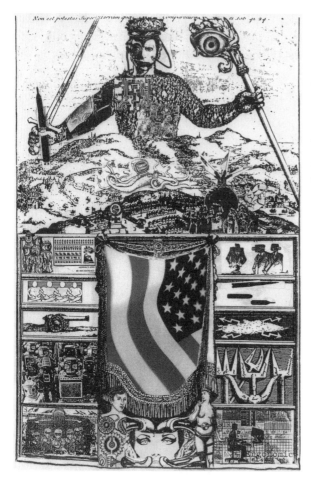

Figure 3. *The Cyborg Body Politic,* collage © Chris Hables Gray.
Society is indeed a monster now, but it is a cyborg and there is no King. The front piece of Hobbes' *Leviathan,* the looming monarch embodied by his people, armed with sword and scepter, with the icons of modern power, is here modified by the author to reflect today's cyborg body politic and the postmodern order.

low the cyborg epistemology proposed in 1995 by myself, Steven Mentor, and Heidi Figueroa-Sarriera: Thesis, Antithesis, Prosthesis, Synthesis. And again. In other words, part of the dynamic is dialectical. As the monetization of culture overwhelmed so much in the twentieth century, attempts were made to limit capital's dominance in the form of anti-monopoly legislation, lobbyist limitations, and campaign finance reform. That these efforts have totally failed has created deeper critiques, especially those of the 21st century movement of movements. They have led directly to open source software, decentralized networking strategies, DIY (do it yourself) projects from the global (indymedia, Linux, Wikileaks, the Social Forum and counter-forum network) to the most local. This nexus of theory is also based on a long practice of grassroots democracy, affinity groups and consensus, feminist process and real community. But other alternative knowledge systems can make use of the same tropes.

Al Queda ("the net" in Arabic) is a perfect example, with its cyborg suicide systems, decentralized command and control with media linkages, a seductive "counter" culture and high levels of secrecy. It is also a reflection in an asymmetrical (as in war) mirror of the information-intensive high-tech cyborg combat systems of the U.S. and NATO and the contrasting liberatory potential of the interweb (Gray 1997, 2005). Reaction, inheritance, prosthesis, reflection, and always something new – the causality of culture is never simple, binary, or ever fully understood.

Human biological evolution in the last 10,000 years has been rapid. Human cultural evolution in the last 10,000 years has been much faster. The relationship between biological, technological, and cultural change is impossible to sort out – but we can certainly affect it. We are it. Emotionally accepting that is the hard part. Coming to terms with our cyborgization is learning how to live with our uncanny feelings, and grow through them. We see this in culture with new belief systems and institutions. But the danger there is believing totally in partial stories. Better to believe partially in many things. And the related danger is to believe in one person, or one small group, to make everything right. It is a system problem.

Knowledge is power and who gets to deploy it is continually being contested. New technoscientific programs are crucial realms for democratizing society since they aren't "locked-in" (Lanier 2010) through technological momentum and because they are sites of cultural and technological production, which is an important form of power. Science and technology in the early 21st century are mainly shaped by market (profit) and military priorities. The sooner new discoveries and inventions can be utilized, the greater their advantage, so incredible resources are poured into those new areas of research that promise maximum returns financially and in military utility. Sometimes within these new areas, resistance to these pressures produces new ways of understanding how science and technology should be in human culture, if they are to help us survive. This seems to be the case with cyborg research, which is becoming a central focus of a wide range of social interventions beyond military contracts and venture capital, such as those mentioned above. And there is art.

There is a longstanding and ongoing discussion of cyborgization in science fiction. But just as important is the growing body of art that engages the "corporeal human-technology convergence" (Borst 2009). It is the human imagination that shapes our future, nothing unimagined comes into being.

Most striking among the cyborg artists are those, such as Stelarc and ORLAN, who take control of their own cyborgization and thus prefigure a democratic technics (Gray 2001).

There is also a resilient movement of scientists and activists that ranges from older groups (the Federation of Atomic Scientists and the Pugwash Network) to newer institutions such as the Loka Institute. In some places citizen juries evalu-

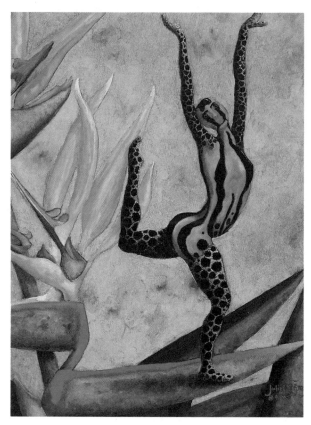

Figure 4. *Petite Paradise*, oil painting © Julia C.R. Gray. The posthuman lives already in the imaginary real. Painting in Alta California, on the edge of the great Pacific Ocean, it is natural that the artist Julia Gray imagines a future with graceful creatures adapted to water and at home in colorful, thriving forests of flowers.

ate the implementation of new technologies, especially medical interventions. As Jenny Reardon shows in her account of the Human Genome Diversity Project, *Race to the Finish* (2004), the making of science is very difficult, and political; and even when scientists are committed to social justice, it doesn't mean their work will be embraced by the populations they are studying, or even trying to help. So the role of citizen groups, which include science academics and scientists themselves, such as The Center for Genetics and Society in California and the Genomics Forum in Scotland, are necessary if technosciences such as genetic engineering are going to be developed with social good as a key criterion, instead of just profit and military advantage as is so often the case.

Two Danish researchers, active in the crucial area of teaching engineers and scientists to consider the ethical and social implications of their work, Andrew Jamison and Niels Mejlgaard, describe the fostering of a "hybrid imagination" that involves "mixing scientific-technical skills with a sense of social responsibility or global citizenship" and where "science and engineering are to help solve social problems rather than create new ones" (2010: 351). This is a crucial part of Cyborg

Citizenship, and when combined with engaged artists and an involved and educated general public, the possibilities of a socially conscious and libratory technoscience begin to emerge.

The growing interweb of internet, telecommunications, social and other new media is integral to this process as well, from intensifying networking and coordination of alternatives to today's world order, to more direct challenges to its truth regime such as Wikileaks. These social initiatives represent a refiguring of knowledge production and control. They reveal how the development of cyborg interventions can lead not just to new inventions and medical treatments, but to stronger democracy as well.

We evolved as social animals. That some people seriously claim that society doesn't exist, that only individuals matter in politics, that only individuals matter in evolution, is absurd. We make politics together; we evolve together. Participatory evolution isn't an individual choice, it is social. It may not be conscious, it may not be considered, and in the past it certainly hasn't been. But today, with the power we have to shape our own genetics, with the understanding we have of how evolution works, and with the warning signs on the horizon that the very nature we are part of is under dire stress and our survival as a species is in doubt, it is time to put selfish illusions behind us and take evolution, and ourselves, seriously.

■ References

Anderson, Stephen and David Lightfoot. 2002. *The Language Organ: Linguistics as Cognitive Physiology*. Cambridge, UK: Cambridge University Press.

Anderson, Walter Truett. 1996. *Evolution Isn't What It Used to Be: The Augmented Animal and the Whole Wired World*. New York: Freeman.

Borst, Elizabeth. 2009. *Cyborg Art: An Explorative and Critical Inquiry into Corporeal Human-Technology Convergence*. Dissertation, University of Waikato, New Zealand.

Brunner, John. 1975. *Shockwave Rider*. New York: Del Rey.

Channell, David. 1991. *The Vital Machine: A Study of Technology and Organic Life*. Oxford: Oxford University Press.

Chorost, Michael. 2005. *Rebuilt: How Becoming Part Computer Made Me More Human*. New York: Houghton-Mifflin.

Clark, Andy. 2003. *Natural-Born Cyborgs: Minds, Technologies and the Future of Human Intelligence*. Oxford: Oxford University Press.

Cochran, Gregory and Henry Harpending. 2009. *The 10,000 Year Explosion: How Civilization Accelerated Human Evolution*. New York: Basic Books.

Diamond, Emma. 2010. 'The Uncanny Valley', http://www.cyborgdb.org.

Dyson, George. 1998. *Darwin Among the Machines: The Evolution of Global Intelligence*. Helix Books.

Editors, 2010. 'Opinion', in *San Francisco Chronicle*, September 12 2010, E10.

Edwards, Paul. 1995. *The Closed World*. Cambridge, MA: MIT Press.

Ehrenrich, Barbara. 1997. *Blood Rites: Origins and History of the Passions of War*. New York: Owl Books.

Flora, Carlin. 2010. 'Why We Share – Interview with Michael Tomassello', in *Discover: Origins*, Summer, 46-7.

Freud, Sigmund. 1919. 'The Uncanny', in *The Complete Works of Sigmund Freud*, London: The Hogarth Press, reprinted in Bruce Grenville, ed. (2001), *The Uncanny: Experiments in Cyborg Culture*, Vancouver Art Gallery, 59-94.

Fukyama, Francis. 2002. *Our Posthuman Future*. New York: Ferrar Straus & Giroux.

Garreau, Joel. 2005. *Radical Evolution: The Promise and Peril of Enhancing Our Minds, Our Bodies – and What it Means to Be Human*. New York: Doubleday.

Gray, Chris Hables. 1997. *Postmodern War: The New Politics of Conflict*. New York: Guilford, London: Routledge.

Gray, Chris Hables. 2001. *Cyborg Citizen*. New York: Routledge.

Gray, Chris Hables. 2005. *Peace, War and Computers*. New York: Routledge.

Gray, Chris Hables et al. 2010. The Cyborg Database, http://www.cyborgdb.org.

Gray, Chris Hables, S. Mentor and H. Figueroa-Sarriera, eds. 1995. *The Cyborg Handbook*. New York: Routledge.

Grenville, Bruce. 2001. 'The Uncanny: Experiments in Cyborg Culture' in *The Uncanny: Experiments in Cyborg Culture*, ed. Bruce Grenville, 13-48, Vancouver Art Gallery.

Haraway, Donna. 1985. 'A Cyborg Manifesto: Science, Technology, and Socialist Feminism in the 1980s', originally published in *Socialist Review*, republished in Haraway 1989.

Haraway, Donna. 1995. 'Cyborgs and Symbionts: Living Together in the New World Order', in *The Cyborg Handbook*, eds. C.H. Gray, S. Mentor and H. Figueroa-Sarriera, xi-xx. New York: Routledge.

Haraway, Donna. 2003. *The Companion Species Manifesto: Dogs, People, and Significant Otherness*. Chicago: Prickly Paradigm Press.

Hard, Mikael and Andrew Jamison. 2005. *Hubris and Hybrids – a Cultural History of Technology and Science*. New York: Routledge.

Harvey, David. 1990. *The Condition of Postmodernity: An Inquiry into the Conditions of Cultural Change*. Cambridge, MA: Blackwell.

Hughes, James. 2004. *Citizen Cyborg*. Boulder, CO: Westview.

Jamison, Andrew and Niels Mejlgaard. 2010. 'Contextualizing Nanotechnology Education: Fostering a Hybrid Imagination in Aalborg, Denmark', in *Science as Culture*, vol. 19, no. 3, 351-368.

Lanier, Jaron. 2010. *You Are Not a Gadget: A Manifesto*. New York: Knopf.

Mann, Steve. 2001. *CYBORG: Digital Destiny and Human Possibility in the Age of the Wearable Computer*. Toronto: Doubleday Canada.

Mazlish, Bruce. 1993. *The Fourth Discontinuity: The Co-Evolution of Humans and Machines*. New Haven: Yale University Press.

Mentor, Steven. 2010. 'The Coming of the Mundane Cyborgs', in *Tecknokultura* (on-line).

Mirowski, Philip. 2002. *Machine Dreams: Economics Becomes a Cyborg Science*. Cambridge: Cambridge University Press.

Morris, Desmond. 1980. *The Naked Ape*, New York: Laurel.

Potts, Malcolm and Thomas Hayden. 2008. *Sex and War: How Biology Explains Warfare and Terrorism and Offers a Path to a Safer World*. Dallas: BenBella Books.

Reardon, Jenny. 2004. *Race to the Finish: Identity and Governance in an Age of Genomics*. Princeton: Princeton University Press.

Sarmiento, Esteban. 2007. *The Last Human: A Guide to Twenty-Two Species of Extinct Humans*. New Haven: Yale University Press.

Scolve, Richard. 1995. *Democracy and Technology*. New York: Guilford.

Stock, Gregory. 1993. *Metaman: The Merging of Humans and Machines into a Global Superorganism*. New York: Simon & Schuster.

Taylor, Timothy. 2010. *The Artificial Ape: How Technology Changed the Course of Human Evolution*. New York: Macmillan.

Teilhard de Chardin, Pierre. 2004. *The Future of Man*. New York: Image.

Toffler, Alvin. 1970. *Future Shock*. New York: Bantam.

Wrangham, Richard. 2009. *Catching Fire: How Cooking Made Us Human*. New York: Basic Books.

Wrangham, Richard and Dale Peterson. 1996. *Demonic Males: Apes and the Origins of Human Violence*. New York: Mariner Books.

■ Acknowledgements

This essay has a complicated genealogy. It is based on my previous writings on cyborgs and several ongoing research projects, such as the Cyborg Database, but its specific origin is a talk in the summer of 2009, "Only Good and Evil: Postmodern Technoscience" at the Belles Artes, Madrid, Spain, sponsored by Cibersomosaguas. I added the idea of the uncyborgable later, when it was put forward by the organizers of Amber '09, a wonderful conference on Art and Technology in Istanbul. This formed the basis for a short article I wrote for the magazine *Literal*, published in Spanish and English. That article was the frame for my keynote talk at the Amber '09 conference and, in turn, parts of both were incorporated into a longer essay for the Amber '09 proceedings, "Uncyborgable", which also drew on an essay written with Steven Mentor, "Cyborgs, Masculinidad, Manifiestos y Cambio Social" published in 2008 in Spanish in *Cultura digital y movimientos socials*, Igor Sabada y Angel Gordo, eds., Madrid: Catarata, pp. 125-148. In July of 2010 I used much material from these to write a long essay, "The Uncanny Evolution of the Cyborg", for a volume being put together by the Contemporary Art Museum of Kaliningrad, Russia, called *Evolution Haute Couture: Art and Science in the Post-Biological Age*. It should be published in Russian and English some time in 2011. Then I rewrote the text again, added illustrations, and changed perspective, and it became "Homo Cyborg: Fifty Years Old" and appears on-line now in *Tecknokultura*. That text has been truncated, modified, and elaborated upon here. In particular I introduce the ideas of cyborg evolution and shockwave riders, and link them to the possibilities of human survival and the probability of sustainable posthumanities.

2 How Close Are We to Being Able to Achieve the Transhumanist Vision?

Maxwell J. Mehlman

Transhumanists look forward to a future in which our descendants have been biologically engineered to be far superior to us. Simon Young predicts, for example, that "humans will complete their evolution from the Stone Age, through the Iron and Industrial ages, to the DNAge, defined by the ability to manipulate human life itself ..." (Young 2006: 37). According to Young, humans must seize this opportunity because they have "The Will to Evolve", and they must not be fainthearted. "Let us cast away cowardice", Young exhorts, "and seize the torch of Prometheus with both hands".

Although the endpoint Young and his fellow transhumanists envision is transcendent, they understand that progress will be gradual; indeed it must be, they concede, so that people can become accustomed to the powerful new biological tools at their command. Transhumanists also accept that evolutionary engineering will begin by targeting disease. According to transhumanist James Hughes, "the first beneficiaries of these technologies will be the sick and disabled, for there is little controversy that they should be able to use technology to more fully control their own lives" (Hughes 2004: 11-12). Nor will all diseases be targeted at once, says Princeton molecular biologist Lee Silver:

> It will begin in a way that is most ethically acceptable to the largest portion of society, with the treatment of only those childhood diseases like sickle cell anemia and cystic fibrosis that have a severe impact on quality of life. The number of parents who will desire this service will be tiny, but their experience will help to ease society's trepidation. (Silver 1997: 237-238)
>
> Gene therapy for serious childhood diseases will be followed by genetic treatments for diseases that are less severe for children or that do not manifest symptoms until adulthood, such as predispositions to obesity, diabetes, heart disease, asthma, and some forms of cancer. (Silver 1997: 237-238; Garreau 2005: 7-8)

After conquering physical disease, transhumanists intend for genetic engineering to turn its attention to mental ailments. Microsoft computer scientist Ramez Naam predicts that ADHD, bipolar disorder, depression, and anxiety will soon fall to the assault of the gene doctors (Naam 2005: 55). Lee Silver adds alcoholism to this list, and Gregory Stock suggests drug addiction. James Hughes predicts that "between gene therapies, better drugs and nano-neuro brain prostheses, mental illness will likely join cancer and aging in being completely preventable and controllable by the latter twenty-first century" (Hughes 2004: 47). Why not proceed to correct emotional dysfunction that may fall short of full-blown mental illness, such as nervousness, gloominess, timidity, and lethargy, asks Simon Young (Young 2006: 37).

With humans now both physically and mentally healthy, the next items on the transhumanists' agenda are enhancements. Young foresees that, like the physical diseases that gene therapy will first address, the first traits to be genetically enhanced will be physical characteristics, traits such as strength, stamina, vitality and virility (Young 2006: 37). Physical beauty certainly will be a prime candidate. Another popular type of modification is likely to be the enhancement of athletic performance. Although the products of recombinant DNA engineering are already being used for this purpose by elite competitors, enhancing performance by directly modifying DNA is a more distant prospect for humans, but researchers are having some success with other species. Transhumanists also have few qualms about enhancing humans by giving them animal genes. Julian Savulescu sees no reason, for example, why people couldn't develop the visual acuity of hawks (Savulescu 2009: 213-214). Enhancing physical abilities will be followed by mental enhancements. Transhumanists expect that genetic modifications will make us more intelligent, give us better memories, and ramp up our powers of concentration. They go beyond improving memory and cognition, however. Silver wants to engineer the mind to make people better at business, art, and music. Stock, noting that "gene therapy has been used to turn lazy monkeys into workaholics by altering the reward centre in the brain" (Stock 2002: 213), wants to enhance industriousness and speculates that perfect pitch may be just a matter of altering a single gene (Stock 2002: 63). Joel Garreau says that we'll do away with the need to sleep (Garreau 2005: 7-8). Stock also predicts that genetic engineering will establish the person's sexual orientation (Stock 2002: 105). Ramez Naam believes that genetic modification will make us friendly, romantic, daring, and empathetic (Naam 2005: 55).

But future humans who are merely healthy, strong, brilliant, and blissful will not have attained transhumanism's ultimate goal. In addition, they will be able to live longer, indeed much longer, perhaps even forever. "The Holy Grail of enhancement", says John Harris, "is immortality" (Harris 2007: 59).

The transhumanists' campaign against death is likely to follow much the same pattern as the other parts of their agenda. Initial efforts will wield genetic engineering as a weapon against the illnesses of old age, and will be passed off as an unremarkable use of gene therapy in the overall battle against disease. This will be followed by more direct attempts to slow or stop the aging process. John Harris predicts that stem cells and other genetic techniques will enable the body to regenerate tissues that are diseased or damaged (Harris 2007: 32-33). Transhumanists find little point in living forever in old bodies, however, even in bodies that remain healthy. So in addition to being immortal, humans will be engineered to be forever young.

How close are we to being able to do these things? Attempts are being made to actively manipulate patients' genes to combat disease, such as the treatments that in 1990 enabled Ashanti DeSilva to develop a partially-functioning immune system. De Silva's treatments were "somatic", however; the altered genes do not reach her eggs and therefore will not be passed on to her children. A more ambitious approach will be germ-line gene therapy, where the corrected genes will be inherited by the patient's children, eradicating the disorder from their descendants.

Until recently, the main way that humans engineered their germ-line was through selective breeding, including the use of mating rituals and more recently, computerized dating services and in vitro fertilization coupled with genetic testing, which allows parents to select desirable genetic characteristics from among those found in their eggs or sperm or in eggs or sperm from donors. But the amount of evolutionary change that PGD makes possible is relatively limited, since it is essentially "passive", in the sense that the parents are choosing which embryos to implant based on the naturally-occurring sets of genes that the embryos have inherited. Plant and animal breeders, on the other hand, have gone beyond passive genetic engineering to employ "active" genetic engineering techniques, such as recombinant DNA, to produce plants and animals that do not occur in nature.

Germ-line genetic engineering has never been attempted deliberately in humans, but it does take place accidentally. A case in point is oocyte transfer, in which a deficiency in an egg that prevents it from successfully developing in the womb is repaired by injecting into it cellular material taken from a normal egg provided by another woman. What makes this qualify as germ-line genetic engineering is that the cellular material from the other woman's egg contains genes from that woman; even though the cellular matter that is inserted comes from outside the cell nucleus, where most of the genes are located, some genes are found in structures outside the nucleus called mitochondria. As a result, a child born from the repaired egg will inherit genes from three people instead of from the normal two: the genes in the father's sperm, the mother's egg nucleus, and the mitochondria in the donor cytoplasm, and this modification will be passed onto this individual's children.

The key question is how hard it would be to produce human germ-line changes intentionally. One approach would be to remove DNA from the nucleus of one of the cells in an embryo fertilized in the laboratory, use gene splicing to modify the DNA, put the DNA back into the cell nucleus, and then stimulate the cell to make it begin to divide normally. If this were done early enough in the development of human embryos, the changed DNA would show up in all of the cells of the resulting persons, including their eggs or sperm, and would therefore be passed on to their children as well. Another approach that has been suggested is to construct an artificial chromosome, embed the modified DNA in it; and inject the chromosome into an embryo cell.

Even if we learn the basic techniques for modifying human germ cells, however, this does not mean that the modifications would be successful. Even though genetic engineering in humans so far has been much less ambitious than what has been done with animals, there have been some noteworthy failures. The most well-known death from a gene therapy experiment was that of 18-year-old Jesse Gelsinger, who died in 1999. Gelsinger was a subject in an experiment at the University of Pennsylvania to develop a genetic treatment for a genetic disease called ornithine transcarbamylase (OTC) deficiency. OTC affects one out of every 40,000 births. Its victims' livers do not produce an enzyme that enables the body to metabolize ammonia, which is a by-product of the breakdown of protein. Affected newborns fall into a coma within 72 hours of birth and suffer severe brain damage. Within a month, half are dead; six months later, 75 percent. Gelsinger himself did not have a full-fledged version of the disease. Instead he had what is termed a "mosaicism" – only some of his liver cells were unable to manufacture the missing enzyme. Gelsinger was fortunate to survive without suffering brain damage, and he was able to control his disease by eating a non-protein diet and taking enzyme pills. But by the time he enrolled in the experiment, he was up to 35 pills a day, and the dosage was bound to have to be increased as time went on. So Gelsinger was keen to serve as an experimental subject, eager to find a cure for himself as well as for the more seriously-affected babies.

The experiment that Gelsinger participated in is what is called a "Phase I" trial. The researchers eventually hoped to insert functional genes into the livers of OTC patients that would enable them to make the enzyme; but first they had to find out if the virus that they proposed to use as the vehicle or "vector" to carry the genes to the liver would get them where they needed to go and in good enough shape to do their job. The experiment was also designed to identify the "maximum tolerated dose" of the treatment – that is, the highest amount of the vector-plus-modified-DNA that could be used without producing serious side effects. The important thing was that the researchers did not expect to actually treat or cure Gelsinger's illness. For their vector, the Penn scientists chose one of the standard ones in use, adenovirus, the virus (actually, a retrovirus) that causes the common cold. Originally, the researchers proposed to use severely-affected newborns as their subjects, but they consulted Arthur Caplan, a leading bioethicist at Penn, who persuaded them to use adults like Gelsinger instead, since they would be better able to give voluntary informed consent to serve as subjects than parents of dying babies (Harris 2007:

31-32). There were 18 subjects in all, divided into groups that would receive different dosages. Gelsinger was in the highest dosage group.

During the night after his infusion, Gelsinger began feeling ill and running a fever, but the doctors weren't alarmed, since other subjects had experienced the same side effects. But Gelsinger's condition continued to deteriorate. He lapsed into a coma, and four days later, he died of massive organ failure (Harris 2007: 31-32).

Two months later, the FDA inspected the research operation at Penn. The agency found fault with the informed consent process that the Penn researchers had used, and determined that Gelsinger should not have been a subject because his liver was not functioning properly when he was given the infusion. In 2005, the Justice Department settled a lawsuit against the Gelsinger researchers in which they were accused of making false statements to the FDA. Their institutions paid over a million dollars in fines, twice the funding they had received from NIH to run the experiment. Gelsinger's father also filed a civil suit, which eventually was also settled.

Gelsinger's death illustrates not only the risks of human genetic experimentation, but the ways in which economic conflicts of interest may make researchers less careful than they should be. The experiment in which Gelsinger died was part of a program at the University of Pennsylvania's Institute of Gene Therapy, which was at the time the largest university program in gene therapy research in the country. The director, James M. Wilson, was also the founder and a stockholder, along with the university, in Genovo, a company that had the exclusive right to profit from any of the institute's discoveries. By the terms of the settlement with the Justice Department, Wilson was barred from conducting FDA-related research on human subjects until 2010.

Another well-known incident involving gene therapy was an effort by French geneticists in 2000 to insert corrected genes into the bone marrow of babies born with a genetic condition that prevented them from developing an immune system. The attempt seemed successful; the babies' immune systems began to function perfectly, and this was heralded as the first complete gene therapy cure. Shortly afterwards, however, three of the children developed leukemia, a form of cancer. It turned out that the retrovirus that the researchers had used to carry the corrected genes into the children's DNA had inadvertently implanted itself too close to a cancer-causing gene, thereby activating it.

Why is genetic engineering so difficult? One reason is that genetics is full of surprises. Until a decade ago, scientists believed that there were approximately 100,000 genes in human DNA, only to find out that the number was closer to 25,000. How could so few genes account for such a complicated organism as a human being? For that matter, how could a tiny member of the cabbage family called thale cress, the first plant to have had its DNA decoded, turn out to possess roughly the same number of genes as humans? The explanation, discovered only recently, is that the same gene can perform many different functions, depending on where and when it is turned on and off. The controls are a set of genetic switches, known as "transcription factors" and "enhancers". These switches are located in the long stretches of the DNA molecule that lie between the genes. Until a few years ago, these regions of DNA were called "junk DNA" because we were certain that they did not play any functional role. Now, geneticists who are conducting "genome-wide association studies", in which they scan the DNA of many in order to identify common variations associated with various traits, are finding 80 percent of these genetic variations in the so-called "regulatory" DNA between the genes (Manolio 2010: 166-176).

Like most things involving genetics, this switching system is extraordinarily complex. Not only can genes be switched on and off, but the functions of a single gene can be affected by many different switches. To gain an idea of just how complex this is, consider this: In order for a gene to work, that is, to produce a protein, one of the things that has to happen is that an enzyme called polymerase has to trigger something called a core promoter, located in the regulatory region next to the gene. The core promoter converts or "transcribes" the DNA in the gene into a substance called messenger RNA. The production of polymerase in turn is controlled by a series of "enhancers" and "silencers". These are sometimes located in far distant regions of the DNA molecule, and each of them can affect a number of different genes. The enhancers and silencers influence the production of polymerase through the actions of large groups of proteins called "activators" and "repressors", which are relayed through another set of proteins called "coactivators" and "basal factors". As many as fifty different proteins may be involved in this process of transcription, all produced by different genes, with each protein individually triggered by a similar complex set of processes (Mayr 2001). Still with me? Now consider that this is only one of many steps that have to take place for a gene to do its work.

The ability of the same gene to perform many functions is called pleiotropy, and it is one of the main reasons why it may be perilous to modify human genes. A mistake not only would impact the particular trait being targeted, such as a genetic disorder, but all the other traits that are associated with that gene. Mistakes are likely to be particularly dangerous when they occur in the course of adding a gene to supplement the functioning of a normal gene by making more of an existing protein, as opposed to being introduced to provide a protein that is missing because of a defective gene. As explained by W. French Anderson, the geneticist who performed the first successful gene therapy experiment on Ashanti DeSilva described earlier, adding protein "might adversely affect numerous other biochemical pathways. In other words, replacing a faulty part is different from trying to add something to a normally-functioning, technically complex system" (Anderson 1989: 686).

Even merely trying to correct a genetic malfunction may produce untoward results if we do not understand enough about how genes work. The classic example is the genetic error that causes sickle cell disease. The error is a single incorrect nucleotide (the basic building blocks of DNA) amid the 3 billion that make up the entire human genetic code. If geneticists were able to cut out the incorrect nucleotide and substitute the correct one in a viable embryonic cell, they might be able to prevent a child who developed from that embryo from being afflicted with sickle cell disease. But in parts of Africa, the sickle cell trait provides resistance to malaria, and this resistance would be lost. The link between the sickle cell mutation and malaria was discovered over 50 years ago, but undoubtedly other "bad" genes confer as-yet unknown benefits that might be forsaken if the genes were removed from human DNA. One commentator wonders, for example, what would happen if any "intellectually desirable attributes are also transmitted with the complex of genes responsible for schizophrenia" (Lappé 1972: 421).

Scientists who nevertheless are keen to try their hand at genetic engineering argue that the discovery of genetic switches provides the solution to the problem of pleiotropy. To avoid upsetting all of the functions associated with a gene, they propose modifying only the switches that affect the targeted trait, not the gene itself (Lappé 1972: 421). But given the intricacies of the switching mechanism, it is not clear how easy this would be to accomplish. Bioethicist Nicholas Agar even thinks trying to reengineer the switching system could end up restoring much of the randomness in natural evolution that genetic engineering is designed to counteract. "Changes to imperfectly understood complex systems", he observes, "produce effects that, relative to our knowledge, are random". Moreover, random changes are not neutral in terms of their effect on an organism: "Random changes to complex, well-functioning systems". notes Agar, "are much more likely to make them work worse than better" (Agar 2004: 162).

Recently, geneticists have also begun to understand that environmental factors, such as diet, exposure to damaging substances, stress, activity, and nurturing not only play a large role in health and behavior, but can also affect whether and to what extent genes are turned on or off in specific tissues, a phenomenon known as "epigenetics" (a field of evolutionary biology that calls itself "evo-devo" emphasizes the importance of epigenetic effects during the early stages of the development of an organism). In other words, environmental factors can modify the functioning of genetic switches, and as a result, tinkering with the switches themselves may not produce the intended effect due to unfavorable conditions in the environment. In addition, there is evidence that epigenetic effects can be inherited (Rothstein et al. 2009:7). Therefore, any errors introduced by a misalignment of environmental factors and intentional action may be passed on to future generations.

Genetic engineering, in short, is incredibly risky. Those at immediate risk of harm are the children whose genes are the subject of such engineering; but their parents may also be affected. For example, greater intelligence in animals is associated with larger brains, and so it is possible that increasing intelligence in humans would expand our brains, and correspondingly, require us to have bigger heads to hold them. Nick Bostrom and Anders Sandberg actually seem to advocate this, envisioning "interventions that moderately increased brain growth during gestation". (Bostrom and Sanderberg 2009: 383). But giving babies bigger heads could prove hazardous during the birthing process as infants with enlarged heads tried to make their way down the birth canal. The problem stems from the fact that the way humans deliver babies is the result of a highly imperfect evolutionary compromise. On the one hand, our brains, and hence our heads, are larger than those of other primates. On the other hand, the human birth canal is shorter and narrower than in other primates in order to strengthen the pelvis so that it can support an upright posture. This produces what some have called the "obstetric dilemma" (Weiner et al. 2008: 469-478). For one thing, in order to get their big brains (and shoulders) through the narrow pelvic passage, human infants must rotate themselves, and so they exit face down, in contrast to other primate babies, which are born face-up. The result is that, whereas other primate mothers can grasp the newborn as it exits and lift it to suckle, it is almost impossible for human mothers to give birth without the assistance of someone else to catch and reposition the baby. In addition, the contest between head size and pelvic shape makes the human birthing process much more painful and dangerous than in other primates. One researcher at the State University of New York at Stony Brook estimates, for example, that between 20% and 25% of all human births have ended in the death of the mother or the fetus (Abitbol 1996). The toll would be much greater except that human babies are born "prematurely" compared to apes and monkeys – 17 months earlier in terms of development than chimpanzees, for example (Mayr 2001: 248-249). Otherwise, babies' heads would be even larger. One response to the obstetric dilemma is to deliver babies surgically via cesarean section, which now accounts for 30% of all U.S. births. Surgical delivery has risks of its own, however, including infections, unplanned hysterectomies, and embolisms (Denk and Aveni 2009). These risks are bound to be reduced with medical progress, and genetic engineers might even be able to refashion human pelvic development so that natural births become easier; but the point remains that genetically modifying one trait may require a cascade of other changes, each with its own set of dangers and unforeseen consequences.

Finally, even if the genetic engineering that is at the heart of the transhumanist agenda could be accomplished safely and effectively, the transhumanists' quest for evolutionary transcendence would still offend religious conservatives. For example, the former chair of President Bush's Council on Bioethics, Leon Kass, is worried that radical changes in human beings would conflict with God's design: "Most of the given bestowals of nature have their given species-specified natures: they are each and all of a given *sort* ... We need more than generalized appreciation for nature's gifts. We need a particular regard and respect for the special gift that is our own given nature" (Kass 2003). Bill McKibben, the author of *Enough!*, argues that using genetics to improve the human race violates our religious heritage. "In the Western tradition", McKibben explains, "the idea of limits goes right back to the start, to a God who made heaven and earth, beast and man, and then decided that it was enough, and *stopped*" (McKibben 2004: 209).

What is especially ironic about the hostility between religious conservatives and transhumanists is that transhumanism can be considered as a techno-religion. Like other religions, it seeks to provide hope in the face of death, a measure of control over the savage aspects of nature, and meaning to its followers' existence. Moreover, the endpoint of humanity that transhumanists envision – eternal life in a blessed state of health and well-being – is strikingly similar to the visions of paradise at the heart of most of the world's religions. The main difference is that religious believers expect to attain paradise if they follow the dictates of their faiths, while with the possible exception of those who arrange to have their bodies or at least their heads cryogenically preserved when they die and therefore might be revived after enormous technological advances have taken place, today's transhumanists cannot hope to enter into their paradise. Yet this may make them all the more insistent on sparing their descendants the same fate.

■ References

Abitbol, Martine M. 1996. *Birth and Human Evolution: Anatomical and Obstetrical Mechanics in Primates*. Westport CT: Bergin & Garvey.

Agar, Nicholas. 2004. *Liberal Eugenics: In Defense of Human Enhancement*. Malden, MA: Blackwell Publishing.

Anderson, W. French. 1989. 'Human gene therapy: why draw a line?', in *Journal of Medicine and Philosophy*, 14: 681-93.

Bostrom, Nick and Anders Sandberg. 2009. 'The Wisdom of Nature: An Evolutionary Heuristic for Human Enhancement', in *Human Enhancement*, eds. Julian Savulescu and Nick Bostrom. Oxford: Oxford University Press.

Denk, Charles E. and Kathryn P. Aveni. 2009. 'Surveillance of Maternal Peripartum Complications Following Cesarean Section'. New Jersey 1997-2005, New Jersey Department of Health and Senior Services. (www.nj.gov/health/fhs/professional/documents/maternal_complications_following_cesarean.pdf) (last visited April 7, 2010).

Garreau, Joel. 2005. *Radical Evolution: The Promise and Peril of Enhancing Our Minds, Our Bodies – and What It Means to Be Human*. New York: Doubleday.

Harris, John. 2007. *Enhancing Evolution: the ethical case for making better people*. Princeton: Princeton University Press.

Hughes, James. 2004. *Citizen Cyborg: Why Democratic Societies Must Respond to the Redesigned Human of the Future*. Cambridge MA: Westview Press.

Kass, Leon. 2003. 'Ageless Bodies, Happy Souls: Biotechnology and the Pursuit of Perfection', in *The New Atlantis*, 1.

Lappé, Marc. 1972. 'Moral obligations and the fallacies of "genetic control"', in 33 (3) *Theological Studies*: 411- 27.

Manolio, Teri A. 2010. 'Genomic Medicine: Genomewide Association Studies and Assessment of the Risk of Disease', in *New Eng. J. Med.*, 363 (2): 166-176.

Mayr, Ernst. 2001. *What Evolution Is*. New York: Basic Books.

McKibben, Bill. 2004. *Enough. Staying Human in an Engineered Age*. New York: Owl Books.

Naam, Ramez. 2005. *More Than Human: Embracing the Promise of Biological Enhancement*. New York: Broadway Books.

Rothstein, Mark A. et al. Winter 2009. 'The ghost in our genes: legal and ethical implications of epigenetics' in *Health Matrix* 19: 1.

Savulescu, Julian. 2009. 'The Human Prejudice and the Moral Status of Enhanced Beings: What Do We Owe the Gods?', in *Human Enhancement*, eds. Julian Savulescu and Nick Bostrom. Oxford: Oxford University Press.

Silver, Lee M. 1997. *Remaking Eden: Cloning and Beyond in a Brave New World*. New York: Avon Books.

Stock, Gregory. 2002. *Redesigning Humans: Our Inevitable Genetic Future*. New York: Houghton-Mifflin.

Weiner, Stuart et al. 2008. 'Bipedalism and parturition: an evolutionary imperative for cesarean delivery?', in *Clincs in Perinatology* 35 (3): 469-478.

Young, Simon. 2006. *Designer Evolution: A Transhumanist Manifesto*. New York: Prometheus Books.

3 Genetics – It Just Got Personal

Lone Frank

"We have entered the era of consumer genetics", remarked Harvard psychologist Steven Pinker in his 2009 essay *My genes, My self*. And while 'consumer genetics' may sound innocuous and even bland, we are in fact talking about a momentous and game changing development. What is quietly unfolding is a biological parallel to the computer revolution.

Just as computers originally were unwieldy mainframes exclusively accessible to professionals, genetics used to be available to the initiated specialists only. But just as it happened with computers, the technological dikes have burst, prices have fallen dramatically, and genetics is fast becoming something quite ordinary and every day. Something anyone can grapple with, because genetic information is readily and cheaply available to the individual.

The great leap forward in consumer genetics came in 2008, when the masses were invited to the personal genetics party as two companies, the Icelandic de-CODEme and the American 23andMe, both launched the personal so-called gene profile or gene scan. By mailing in a bit of saliva or a cheek swab, you can be tested for between half a million and a million genetic markers. These variants, called single nucleotide polymorphisms or SNPs, are then compared with the results of a number of well-known genetic association studies – studies that have identified SNPs that increase or decrease the risk of a range of illnesses. From cardiovascular disease and diabetes to Alzheimer's and gout.

What you get is not a classic genetic diagnosis informing you that you either have or probably will get a certain disease, but rather a risk assessment. A broad collection of risk indicators of where you are in relation to the general population. For instance, you may turn out to have a 6 or 50 percent statistical risk of developing Alzheimer's some time in your life compared to the average of 12 percent.

The personal gene profile was generally touted in the media worldwide, and was even named invention of the year by *TIME Magazine*. But obviously, this is just the beginning. A first primitive generation of products that will soon seem comparable to PCs like Commodore 64s or the very first Macintosh machines, which now seem ancient to us.

With ever cheaper sequencing technologies emerging, most experts agree that within the next three years a full genome sequence will be available for just 1,000 dollars. Others confidently predict that in ten years' time most newborns will have their full genome mapped and deciphered as a matter of routine. The question then becomes: What will this personal genomics revolution *mean*? Not just for treating and preventing disease, but for our understanding of who we are? In other words: How will genetic information affect our view of ourselves as individuals and of what it is to be human?

Genes of behavior back in fashion

"All human behavioral traits are heritable", dictates the first law of behavioral genetics as famously formulated by University of Virginia psychologist Eric Turkheimer. This means of course that there is a genetic component to all our behavioral traits, a component that varies in size depending on the trait in question, and a component that is in constant negotiation with environmental influences. And judging from the coverage in major scientific journals and the popular media both, the field of behavior genetics is on the ascent (Holden 2008: 892-895).

The interest in how genes play a role in our behavior through affecting our temperament, our psyche and our personality is rising and research projects that would not have been politically possible a few years ago are now being launched. In Europe, for example, there is the IMAGEN project, in which researchers scattered across the continent will follow two thousand teenagers over four years. They will regularly be given a brain scan, be subjected to psychological tests, and fill out questionnaires about their lives and doings. At the same time, they will be tested for a whole battery of genes. *We conduct this study in order to better understand the teenage mind*, the purpose statement says, and the hope is to find some patterns that predict psychological and behavioral problems and to head those problems off through a treatment based on biology.

In fact, a small handful of genes which typically exist in different variations and which impact measurably on aspects of our psyche and temperament are currently known. One is the gene SERT, which encodes the serotonin transporter. A protein which sits embedded in the surface of brain cells capturing the transmitter substance serotonin and sending it back into the cell, after it has been released to provide a signal. One component of the SERT gene is a sort of regulator that determines how much transporter protein is produced. And this regulator is found in a shorter and a longer variant, the shorter one having the effect that less of the transporter protein is manufactured.

The short variant has consistently been linked to a higher score on the personality trait neuroticism. In the now famous Dunedin studies by Avshalom Caspi and Terry

Moffit of Kings College, it has furthermore been associated with an increased risk of developing depression in adult life, but *only* when an individual was exposed to abuse or neglect early in life.

A similar story can be told of the MAOA gene. It codes for the enzyme mono-amine oxidase A, which breaks down a number of transmitter substances such as adrenaline, noradrenaline and serotonin. Less effective variants lead to the production of less or no enzyme and, thus, an overflow of the transmitter substances in areas of the brain. Variants of MAOA have been implicated in "social sensitivity" as well as compulsive gambling and psychiatric conditions such as hyperactivity and obsessive compulsive disorder. Again, the Dunedin studies of Caspi and Moffit have shown that the less effective MAOA variants increase the risk of aggressive and violent behavior in adults who were victims of an abusive childhood.

With these studies in mind, the literature has often termed the less effective variants of both SERT and MAOA "risk" variants. They were seen as variants that conferred psychological vulnerability. But this simple story is now under revision by people such as Jay Belsky, a child psychologist at London's Birckbeck University. Using both his own data and that of other researchers, he has pointed out that carriers of the "risk" variants seem to have a decreased risk of depression, anxiety and violent behavior in the absence of an abusive childhood.

What is conferred by these gene variants is not vulnerability but *susceptibility*. When it comes to genes such as SERT and MAOA, the variants that used to be characterized as "vulnerable" should rather be considered as variants that provide plasticity. Belsky argues that they make the nervous system more sensitive to impressions and, thus, more flexible (Belsky and Pluess 2009: 885-908). Flexibility, in turn, means that with these variants, you are more susceptible not just to negative influences but also, and to the same degree, positive circumstances.

Embracing complexity

If or when we all have our genomes sequenced and displayed for us, how will insights into the genetic underpinnings of our psychological dispositions affect our lives?

"Will 'risk' and 'potential' eventually dominate ideas of personal identity?" ask Ilina Singh and Nikolas Rose in a splashy opinion piece in *Nature*. "And will these ideas become institutionalized within education, law and policy?" (Singh and Rose 2009: 202-207).

The two biologically-conscious social scientists at the London School of Economics would have us discuss what genetic predictions can do to our lives, if they are with us from the beginning. How will it influence parents if they can read about certain risks and potentials in their newborn's gene profile? Will it color their view of their child, and will it change the way they treat the apple of their eye? And what will it do to the child's view of himself that he is labeled from the outset as being at risk, particularly sensitive, robust, or whatever?

Singh and Rose are articulating the fear that purely statistical dispositions may be transformed into self-fulfilling prophecies for the individual simply because we know about them and may begin to behave in conformity with them. And you can easily imagine ugly scenarios in which too heavy-handed expectations crush or lead astray unfortified souls. On the other hand, you can also imagine how some genetic alarm bells may trigger an effort to equip more fragile temperaments with vital defenses. Sensitive souls could be helped if genetics tell us that they are susceptible to positive influence.

One thing is life in the family, but these perspectives reach far beyond the private sphere. Now that this genetic knowledge exists, might some even try and base policies upon it? There are those who believe we can and should. And some would point to a study from 2009 in which a research team led by psychologist Gene Brody of the University of Georgia ventured into territory where few people have dared to go. They selected a group of poor black children, tested them for variants of the SERT gene, and observed their behavior.

The Brody team went way out into the boonies of Georgia, canvassed a poor black community and then selected 641 families, all of which had an 11-year old child. A child that was on the cusp of puberty with all the risks that implies for getting involved with alcohol, drugs and sex – collectively dubbed risk behavior. The researchers wanted to follow the children until they turned 14 and investigate two things: First, whether children with the short SERT variant are particularly predisposed to risk behavior; and, second, whether there is a genetic difference in how children react if those around them are trying to keep them from getting into trouble (Brody et al. 2009: 645-661).

It went like this: the children were gene-tested and divided into two groups of which one was allowed to go their own way, while the other, together with the whole family, entered into a support program called The Strong African American Families Program or SAAF. This is a program that takes parents to school and teaches them to participate in their children's lives, and in particular to set limits for them. And they know that it works. Statistically speaking, the effort has a positive effect on children's risk behavior.

Now, it turned out over the next few years that, in the group that was left to itself, the young people with the short version of SERT began to smoke, drink alcohol, and have sex with twice the frequency of the kids with two copies of the long version. It looked like they were genetically predisposed to throw themselves into risk behavior, an observation that corresponded to the researchers' presumptions.

However, a far more sensational finding had to do with the group that was a part of SAAF. The program had a considerable preventative effect on the "genetically disadvantaged" individuals but only a poor effect on the rest. For both groups, the frequency of risk behavior was pretty much down at the same level as for kids with two long SERT variants who did not participate in SAAF. Intervention clearly worked best for the children who were particularly genetically sensitive. Or, rather, *susceptive*.

What can a finding like this be used for? Undoubtedly, there are those who will cross themselves, get nervous palpitations, and mumble something about stigmatization and social disadvantages. It could also be said that here is some research that speaks directly against the fear that behavior genetics will only point out "bad" genes and be the cause of labeling some group as hopelessly biologically inferior. On the other hand, this genetic research is a direct illustration of the fact that social initiatives pay off where the problems are most dire. It does not necessarily suggest that young children should be routinely subjected to gene-testing and subsequently labeled as more or less suitable for help. Rather, it shows that the very knowledge we get from new genetic studies can shake up our understanding and thus influence policy.

A small group of social scientists is beginning to realize the possibilities, and one of the more interesting is criminologist Nicole Rafter, who published *The Criminal Brain* in 2008. Here, among other things, she goes through the dubious history of biological criminology, its mistakes and its hopelessly unscientific basis. But directly opposed to the reader's expectations, Rafter ultimately came to the conclusion that biological studies in a *modern* context may be good.

"We're *not* talking about more of the same", she underlines. Today's behavior genetics turns the genetic determinism of the past completely upside down, and this has huge implications for research, treatment, policy, and the relationship between researchers.

Rafter speaks warmly in favor of a new "biosocial" thinking, a way of thinking that marries sociological and biological understandings of why people behave the way they do under different circumstances. Biologists must definitively come to terms with the earlier medical mode of thinking, which views behavior – including criminality – as either healthy or sick, normal or abnormal. Social scientists, for their part, must incorporate biological knowledge and thinking into their sociological theories. If that happens, it may be the most effective way to create programs that address criminality by treating social ills. As Rafter provocatively ends her book: "I want to enlist modern genetics in progressive social change".

Can genetics really bear this? Possibly. But it requires a brutal liquidation of some hardy, old myths. And this requires that a more realistic view of what genes are and what they can do becomes more widespread in the population and permeates culture itself. This is no easy task, but there are some handles to grab onto.

One example is the new thinking in psychiatry, where front runners are in the process of tossing out the conception of risk genes in favor of genetically-determined susceptibility. This is an important change in consciousness, as the focus shifts from the risk of an unfortunate outcome to the potential for a good outcome. And this is a potential that is not determined by the genome itself but can only be realized by external circumstances. It is a loud 'no' to classic genetic determinism.

Another necessary readjustment has to do with the idea that the genome is something static. Many people have a rooted sense that because our genes can't be changed, we are in some way or other strapped into a biological straightjacket. But this is where the emerging field of epigenetics acts as a great corrective.

Epi – that elegant, little Greek prefix indicates that we are dealing with something "above" or "beyond" genetics itself. Epigenetics has come to stand for the regulation of the way genes are *expressed* – that is, how much or how little protein they are allowed to produce, at what time, and in what cells. These are changes in the function of genes that occur without mutations in the genetic sequence. They are effectuated by a suite of enzymes which can change the three-dimensional structure of DNA and in that way switch a gene's activity off or on.

With these quirky switches, the genome is suddenly revealed to be something incredibly dynamic. In the last few years epigenetic changes in gene activity have been implied in setting an individual's stress response. Clearly, we are just beginning to scratch the surface of the possibilities for plasticity, but we can already see how information that is in itself immutable is always subject to *interpretation* by different tissues, and that interpretation can make for colossal differences. It is also clear that interpretation can be manipulated – again by all sorts of environmental and external circumstances. The upshot is that the most effective way to shape us human beings is not to change the genes themselves but to change what we subject the genes to.

In fact, the rise of epigenetics will undoubtedly lead to a new and, hopefully, intense interest in the environment in the broadest possible sense. All the indicators point toward the fact that genetic research is increasingly becoming a more holistic investigation of the ever on-going interplay between the genome, the organism, and all those myriad factors that can be termed 'the environment'. In other words, it is opening up the complexity that is the fundamental condition of biology and an inseparable part of its beauty.

From homogeneity to diversity

Dynamism and complexity are key concepts. I predict that, in the future, a third watchword might prove to be *diversity* – in the sense of genetic and, thus, biological and behavioral diversity.

Because in the near future a degree of diversity we never dreamed of is going to come crashing in on us. Researchers will have thousands and, soon, millions of individual genomes to play with, and the exercise will provide fascinating surprises from and new insights into how *different* our genomes are, *how* they are different, and what the difference *means*. We've already had a little foretaste of this diversity with projects that have mapped and compared broad ethnic groups – or races, if you will. There was the international HapMap Project which grew out of the Human Genome Project and used DNA from a handful of individuals to compare certain variations between the major racial groups. Recently, we have been hearing results from The 1000 Genomes Project, which is well on its way to fully sequencing and publishing a thousand genomes belonging to individuals of several ethnicities. But before long we will presumably see genomes from the Bushmen and the Pygmies, from Inuits, Australian aborigines, and everything in between. But also within each of these groups, diversity will unfold in ever more detail and, when it comes down to it, this may be a welcome corrective to the earlier insistence on what was common to human beings.

This has been a mantra in genetic research. In toasts and official statements, it has been said that what is interesting about studying different genomes is discovering how *uniform* they are. The genome has been employed to create a sort of fraternization across cultural, historical, and social differences, and this has been politically motivated. But since we now know perfectly well that we are and will remain one species, it seems completely obvious that what is really exciting is what makes us, despite everything, different from each other in so many ways. As individuals and as groups with different origins.

But, right here, we should prepare ourselves to have a discussion, believe geneticist Bruce Lahn from the University of Chicago and economist Lanny Ebenstein from the University of California, Santa Barbara. In a commentary in *Nature*, they try to start it themselves. It may be, the two point out, that the research will reveal a difference we don't care for. What if it turns out there are genetic differences between population groups that have a biological significance that is politically repulsive? This is utterly conceivable and, therefore, according to Lahn and Ebenstein, we need "a moral response to this question that is robust irrespective of what research uncovers about human diversity". (Lahn and Eberstein 2009: 726-728).

This is courageous. For the two are up against not only historical racial ideology and all its unscientific dictums, but also the more contemporary discussion of the extent to which and, in the given case, why there are average differences in intelligence among population groups. It touched off huge outcry when, in 1995, the book *The Bell Curve* pointed to a so-called 'intelligence gap'. Armed with many years of IQ measurements from a number of countries and populations, authors Richard Herrnstein and Charles Murray concluded that there seems to be a typical pattern of bell curves that describe intelligence in a population. You find the curve for Caucasians in the middle of the field, while blacks are lower and Asians are higher. Not a popular finding. There doesn't seem to be anything to call the curves and the measurements into question, but the debate is about the extent to which the differences are due to genes or reflect purely environmental effects.

One wing of researchers, led by British neurobiologist Steven Rose, argues that you get past the problem by refusing to investigate differences in intelligence at all. Nothing will come from it except quite possibly discrimination if differences are indeed found, maintains Rose (Rose 2009: 786-788).

On the other hand, Lahn and Ebenstein claim that a thorough exploration of genetic diversity – whatever it may bring to light – can act as a medicine against discrimination. Simply because it will make it clear that it is impossible, if not to say ridiculous, to rank groups or individuals by some one-dimensional scale. Genetic diversity contributes to variation across domains – physical and mental. And there is no single measurable trait, such as IQ, that says anything exhaustive about an individual's total mental capacity. As the duo insist:

"We argue for the moral position that genetic diversity, from within or among groups, should be embraced and celebrated as one of humanity's chief assets".

And we love diversity, right? In every possible connection, difference is elevated as a value. Modern society cultivates, talks about and celebrates cultural diversity, and many of us react to globalization's threat of general homogenization by appreciating what is different. That which we don't already know. And as far as nature is concerned, diversity is king. Monoculture is the great sin of industrialized agriculture, and environmentalists are fighting a bitter struggle for biodiversity. To save threatened toads, special corals, obscure bird species, and other living things only the very few ever see. In fact, we find ourselves in the midst of a mass extinction of species on the planet, and biodiversity is well on its way toward becoming the next great topic in environmentalism.

So why not cultivate and protect our own biological diversity? The consciousness that we are a species with characteristic genetic differences and physical variation could be the hook that finally gets us to worry about threatened peoples. Populations whose way of life, cultural peculiarities, and language are on the verge of extinction – along with their special genetic composition. It might be South Africa's ancient San people, the Amazon's diverse Indian peoples, or marginalized populations in the Russian taiga, to mention a few.

Toward a culture of biology

The interest in genetic diversity may even be an entryway to a new understanding of cultural and intellectual diversity. At least, psychologists Matthew Lieberman and Baldwin Way of the University of California at Los Angeles have put forward some interesting ideas about how genetic differences between ethnic groups may help determine where a given culture puts down roots in the world.

The two have contrasted Asian and Western culture. They forget everything about the subtle differences between Japanese and Vietnamese or French and British and focus on a very characteristic difference that is deposited over and above all the specifics – namely, that Eastern Asian culture is collectivist, while we in the West are individualists. For decades, anthropologists have studied and described how this is expressed, but the two psychologists asked *why* this is the case. Is it entirely random, or might there be a biological foundation for the state of things?

They answer with the hypothesis that what is decisive is differences in social sensitivity. And that this difference in sensitivity is ultimately based on the fact that the incidence of the sensitive – or susceptible – variants of a number of specific genes is different in the two cultures.

The idea is grating to many ears, especially to people inclined toward the humanities. But Way and Lieberman have some interesting observations to point to. They have looked at studies of social sensitivity in relation to three selected genes: the by now familiar SERT, MAOA (which encodes the enzyme monoamine oxidase A), and the gene for a receptor found in the brain that is activated by opioids. These three genes are all found in a variant that has been proven to increase sensitivity to social stress, but which also provides a high susceptibility to the beneficial effect of an environment where there is a high degree of social support.

When you study Asian and Caucasian populations, it appears that the frequency of the sensitive variants of all three genes is between two and three times as high in Asian peoples as in Caucasian. And what does this mean, ask Way and Lieberman.

It means that more Asians do better with a high degree of social support and positive social relations – which is best achieved in a collectivist culture, where people are embedded in a strong social network. Therefore, for example, the idea of the Chinese philosopher Confucius that the family and the group is the important thing that the individual must take into consideration has triumphed throughout Asia. By contrast, there are fewer Caucasians who are particularly sensitive to social rejection and exclusion, which is why ideas about the individual's need to take precedence over the community has had an easier time in Europe and the rest of the Western world. As Liebermann writes:

"When enough brains are predisposed to find the same idea compelling, it is likely to stick around for quite some time" (Liebermann 2009).

The two young psychologists have come up with a radical innovation that will certainly raise an outcry from traditional cultural research. One can imagine how vicious accusations about genetic determinism and reductionism of the worst sort will be aired in the pages of professional journals. But the question is whether Way and Lieberman herald a shift in the way we think about human beings. A shift that can be sensed when social scientist James Fowler calls for "a new science of human nature". He says very directly that no human science can explain human behavior and culture without integrating human biology – from genes to brain function (Fowler and Schreiber 2008: 912-914).

All this research and the researchers behind it are moving toward a genuinely biological view of human beings. A view that takes its starting point in what the creature *Homo sapiens* is and whose understanding is based on a knowledge of evolution, genetics and brain physiology. *And* culture and history. It is not about biological man being in opposition to cultural man. The point is a comprehensive understanding that, of course, integrates the products of human behavior and ideas – politics, culture, music, poetry – and considers them in a biological context. And vice versa.

If there is anything that can drive this transformation beyond the academic sanctuary, it is personal genetics. Quite simply because the phenomenon is a teaching device for the individual that works on the individual's premises. Even now, genetic tests can be bought in supermarkets in certain places, and tens of thousands of people around the world are in the process of making an intimate acquaintanceship with genetic information by using it. This is decisive. Because it is only when you get the information in your hands and, so to speak, under your skin that you really experience it and understand its significance.

And there is no doubt that personal access and the personal approach to genetic information has come to stay. It will be developed and get ever more content and detail. Today, it is a million SNPs, tomorrow the whole genome, and the day after the genome with its epigenetic changes in the body's various tissues and organs. Eventually, we won't be able to conceive of ourselves without this information, and it will quite naturally enter into many of our everyday decisions.

Consumer genetics is still largely portrayed to us as a question of disease, health, and prevention – the great goal of it all being personalized medicine tailor-made for our particular genetic make up. Illness is an important matter, we can't get around it, but it is far from the most important. Deep down, an increased genetic consciousness has to do with our self-understanding. Our knowledge of who we are – as a species among other species and as individuals. And finding out about your own DNA invariably has the wonderful effect of raising a lot of major and profound questions.

Who are we? Where do we come from? What is our place in the world? Where are we going? What do we want? These sorts of questions are traditionally delegated to the "spiritual" realm, but when it comes right down to it, they are better answered by digging deeper into the physical reality.

However, if we buy into the biological view of man and increase our genetic consciousness, what will it do to our self-understanding? This, among other things, is what the Canadian philosopher, Ian Hacking, would like to know.

"I'm a conservative reactionary," he admits in an essay on consumer genetics and identity (Hacking 2009).

I know that although my genetic inheritance constrains my possibilities of action and choice, I do not believe it is my essence or constitutes my identity. My question could be put: how long will it take before this attitude becomes extinct? We know that the genomic revolution will radically change the material conditions of life for soon-to-be-born generations. My question is: what will be the conception of self for those people soon to come? (Hacking 2009)

Hacking frets that, from now on, we will have the sense that we *are* our genes in a narrow-minded way. I think he is worrying unnecessarily.

In the course of investigating consumer genetics I have myself become a customer and have entered into a number of available tests, Thus, I have looked deeply into my own genes and reflected on this vision for many months, and the result is not a simplified self-image. On the contrary. It is rather the case that I'm experiencing more facets and nuances. It is far more satisfying to be able to interpret yourself and your life from both a biological and a social and cultural perspective. It becomes very clear that genes are *not* fate but, on the contrary, cards we are dealt, and some cards provide you with a certain latitude in your game. The genome is not a straightjacket but a soft sweater you can fill out and shape. It is information we can work with and, thus, information that can help provide greater freedom to shape our lives and our own essence. On the other hand, it is also information that can, in its way, ease an existential burden. It tells us that we are not totally free, nor are we completely responsible for who we are and what we become.

So who am I? I am what I *do* with this incredible information that has flowed through millions of years through billions of organisms and has finally been entrusted to me.

The text is an edited excerpt of Lone Frank's latest book, *My Beautiful Genome*. Gyldendal 2010, Oneworld Publishers 2011.

■ References

Belsky, Jay and Michael Pluess. 2009. 'Differential susceptibility to environmental influences', in *Psychological Bulletin*, vol. 135 (6): 885-908.

Brody, H. Gene et al. 2009. 'Prevention Effects Moderate the Association of 5-HTTLPR and Youth Risk Behavior Initiation: GeneEnvironment Hypotheses Tested via a Randomized Prevention Design', in *Child Development*, vol. 80 (3): 645-661.

Fowler, James H. and Darren Schreiber. 2008. 'Biology, Politics, and the Emerging Science of Human Nature', in *Science*, vol. 322 (5903): 912-914.

Hacking, Ian. 2009. 'Commercial genome reading' on TheHuman.org. Accessed in March 2011 http://onthehuman.org/2009/03/current-controversies-ian-hacking/.

Holden, Constance. 2008. 'Parsing the Genetics of Behavior', in *Science*, vol. 322: 892-895.

Lahn, Bruce T. and Lanny Ebenstein. 2009. 'Let's celebrate human genetic diversity', in *Nature*, vol. 461 (18): 726-728.

Lieberman, Matthew D. 2009. 'What makes big ideas sticky?', in *What's Next? Dispatches on the Future of Science: Original Essays from a New Generation of Scientists*, ed. Max Brockman. Madison, AL: Vintage.

Rose, Steven. 2009. 'Darwin 200: Should scientists study race and IQ? NO: Science and society do not benefit', in *Nature*, vol. 457: 786-788.

Singh, Ilina and Nikolas Rose. 2009. 'Biomarkers in psychiatry', in *Nature*, vol. 460 (9): 202-207.

4 The Medicine of the Future – Live Long and Prosper?

Søren Holm

Imagine going to the doctor in 25 or 100 years' time. What complaints will the typical patient present their doctor with, and what treatments will be available for those complaints? And, more generally: what will be the implications for the medicine of the future of our current rapid advances in the understanding of human biology and the technological use of that understanding? Will there even be something that is recognisable as medicine, or will the field have changed shape so radically that doctors and hospitals are only distant memories?

This chapter will try to look into the medical crystal ball and predict the medicine of the future. This is not easy, and the longer the time span is the less accurate the specific predictions will be. Everything here should therefore be taken *cum grano salis*. I rarely write texts in which I know that I am wrong, but the present chapter is an exception. I am completely certain that most of the specific predictions I make will be wrong. I can only hope that they are generally right and only wrong in the detail.

What can we learn from past predictions?

Predicting the future progress of medicine is nothing new.[1] Medical doctors have been doing it for thousands of years, philosophers have been in on the act, and futurologists of all kinds have also contributed their predictions.

Let us begin our brief survey of the past of these predictions with a quote from the philosopher René Descartes in his *Discourse on Method* which very nicely encapsulates two features common to many predictions:

> But it was not only my desire for the invention of an infinite number of devices which might enable us to enjoy without effort the fruits of the earth and all the commodities found in

---

1. In the research for this section of the paper I have been immensely helped by the Paleo-Future blog and website http://www.paleofuture.com/.

it, but mainly also my desire for the preservation of our health, which is, without doubt, the principal benefit and the foundation of all the others in this life. For even the mind depends so much on the temperament and the condition of the organs of the body that, if it is possible to find some means to make human beings generally wiser and more skilful than they have been up to this point, I believe we must seek that in medicine. It is true that the medicine now practiced contains few things which are remarkably useful. *But without having any design to denigrate it, I am confident that there is no one, not even those who make a living from medicine, who would not claim that everything we know in medicine is almost nothing in comparison to what remains to be known about it and that we could liberate ourselves from an infinity of illnesses, both of the body and the mind, and also perhaps even of the infirmities of ageing, if we had sufficient knowledge of their causes and of all the remedies which nature has provided for us.* (my emphasis) (Descartes 2010 [1637])

The first feature is the simultaneous lament concerning the present state of medicine ("almost nothing in comparison to what remains to be known"), combined with a promise of a future essentially without illness or ageing. And the second feature is the claim that if we just understood the causes of illness and the available remedies, we could easily bring about the promised future. These two features recur again and again. It is worth noting that although biological casual knowledge is immensely valuable in developing new treatments, it does not in and of itself guarantee that treatments can be developed.

Let us move forward in time to 1900. The dawning of new centuries has always been seen as an appropriate point at which to take stock of the old and predict the new, and in 1900 the chairman of the British Medical Association, John W Byers did exactly that in a Presidential Address:

In thinking over a suitable subject for a presidential address it is only natural that, at the close of a century, the characteristic note of which has been, as stated by Mr. Balfour in his masterly address to the summer meeting of the Cambridge University Extension students, its fertility "in the products of scientific research to which no other period offers a precedent or parallel," one should feel the present occasion would be an admirable opportunity to look backwards and try to answer the question, How has the science and art of medicine in its various departments been influenced by all those wonderful discoveries of this century, which dazzle us not merely by their ingenuity and by the rapidity with which they have followed one another, but still more by their practical application in this most utilitarian age, to the diagnosis, prevention, and treatment of disease? "No century," according to Mr. Balfour, "has seen so great a change in our intellectual appreciation of the world in which we live," and we, from a purely medical point of view, join with him in saying now, "We not only see more but we see differently." Even within the experience of many present to-day, has not the science of bacteriology completely revolutionised our ideas in almost very branch of medicine? And with the last few years a new and most promising field for original investi-gation has been opened up by the combined clinical and laboratory investigations of the blood; and so, at the end of this century, another medical science arises – hæmo-pathology. (Byers 1990: 1363-1366)

What makes Byers' predictions interesting is that he was both right and wrong at the same time. He correctly identified two recent successful research programs, but then based his predictions on only those two. Bacteriology and hæmo-pathology would continue to be important areas of medical development, both scientifically and in relation to clinical practice in the 20th century; but other areas of medicine, unknown to Byers, would become even more important. Many new diseases would be discovered and invented because of new scientific discoveries, and they would all need new remedies. And the great success of the microbial research program would also lead some researchers astray. The Danish pathologist C.J. Salomonsen, for instance, identified the – in his words "dysmorphic" – creations of some modern artists as the result of a new, contagious mental illness (Abildgaard 1984-1985); and the Danish scientist J.A.G. Fibiger was awarded the Nobel Prize in Physiology or Medicine in 1926 for his spurious linkage of cancer to the nematode worm Spiroptera carcinoma.[2]

Predictions in newspapers and other public media are also worth a look. In 1955 the Chairman of the section of general practice of the American Medical Association gave a public address beginning with the declaration that "Medicine has made more progress in the first half of the 20th century than in the 6,000 previous years".[3] He then went on to make 10 predictions for the state of medicine in 1999. I have taken the liberty of only quoting those that are, in retrospect, dubious:[4]

1. A man 90 years old will be considered "young", a man of 135 "more mature" and there will be "a minimum of senility because the heavy cholesterol which determines the age of our arteries will be absent.
2. Our women, thanks to proper hormone medication, will stay young, beautiful and shapely [sic!] indefinitely.[5]
   [...]

---

2. http://nobelprize.org/nobel_prizes/medicine/laureates/1926/. The worm has since been renamed Gongylonema neoplasticum.
3. http://www.paleofuture.com/display/ShowImage?imageUrl=/storage/1955 June 9 Charleston Gazette – Charleston WV paleo-future.jpg?__SQUARESPACE_CACHEVERSION=1246589444798.
4. Other predictions from the 1950s include a prediction in 1958 of the imminent arrival of space hospitals taking advantage of the lack of gravity to provide new and more effective treatments. http://www.paleofuture.com/blog/2009/8/9/hospitals-in-the-sky-1958.html. In 2010 we still have problems servicing a single, multinational space station!
5. This was unsurprisingly the prediction that caught the eye of the headline writer, who ran the story under the headline "'Fountain of Youth' for Womenfolk?".

4. All human infectious disease [...] will be eradicated by "use of vaccines, antibiotics and multiphasic screening tests.
5. Cancer will be successfully treated by a virus vaccine or radioactive compounds.
6. The common cold [...] will be only a memory.[6]
   [...]
8. Synthetic foodstuffs will bring an end forever to famine and starvation.
   [...]
10. Insulin will be given in tablet form for the control of diabetes.

It is not for lack of scientific and clinical effort that these predictions did not come to fruition. Research budgets and numbers of researchers increased at very fast rates between 1955 and 1999. So what went wrong? Irrational exuberance may be part of the explanation, but there are other important factors as well. Prediction number 6, the eradication of the common cold, offers us a good example to tease out some of these factors. Not only is the common cold not eradicated, the symptomatic treatments we have are no better than in 1955. The prediction about the common cold falls within prediction number 4 as a specific subset. Why have we not eradicated the common cold, despite very considerable research efforts? Through research we have identified the causal viral agents and gained large amounts of knowledge about how these viral agents interact with the epithelia of the upper respiratory tract and how they interact with the immune system.[7] So the lack of effective treatment, not to mention treatment so effective that the disease can be eradicated, is not primarily due to lack of knowledge (Tyrell and Fielder 2002). The knowledge generated even put us in a good position to explain why we haven't made the common cold "only a memory". More than 200 viruses can cause the kind of condition we label a 'common cold', so we can't vaccinate against it; and no single drug works against more than a handful of these viruses, so we can't treat it. There is furthermore evidence that vaccination might well be counterproductive, since it is the activation of the immune system that causes many of the symptoms and people who are re-exposed to a specific virus and therefore generate a quick immune response may get a worse cold than those who are exposed for the first time. So the common cold problem is simply very, very complicated and may be one of those medical problems that although solvable in theory are unsolvable in practice. Although the common cold problem initially looks like 'the polio problem' or 'the measles problem', for instance, in being an acute infectious illness caused by a virus, it is in reality completely different.

---

6. While writing this I have one, so can personally vouch for the fact that it is 'not only a memory'!
7. For a fascinating account of the history of common cold research and treatments, see Jennifer Ackerman. Ah-Choo! The Uncommon Life of Your Common Cold. New York: Twelve, 2010.

The first and second predictions made in this talk in 1955 are also interesting. They fall in a long line of predictions of radical changes in longevity and health, and like many such predictions they predicate the claims about the future on a very limited number of factors (in this case cholesterol and hormones). If we can just reduce cholesterol and titrate our hormone treatments appropriately, both men and women will have very long and shapely lifespans. Again, this has not happened 55 years after the prediction was made. A man of 90 is not considered young now; and I confidently predict that when I reach 90 in 43 years time I will not be considered young or shapely.[8] One of the things that has gone wrong here is a very typical mistake in predicting the medical future. The most extensive possible therapeutic promises of one or two recent scientific successes are projected forward and claimed to be reality.

Let us finally move to the most recent predictions. The UK government-sponsored website "sciencesowhat", aimed at making young people interested in the sciences in 2010, predicted some future careers that young people could aim at in 2025. Six of these jobs are in medicine:

1. *Body part maker* Advances in science will make it possible to create living body parts, so we could need living body part makers, body part stores and body part repair shops.
2. *Nano-medic* Advances in nanotechnology for creating molecular-scale devices and treatments could transform personal healthcare so we would need a new breed of nano medicine specialists to administer these treatments.
3. *Pharmer* of genetically engineered crops and livestock. New age farmers will grow crops and keep animals that have been genetically engineered to increase the amount of food they produce and to include proteins that are good for our health. Scientists are already working on a vaccine-carrying tomato and therapeutic milk from cows, sheep and goats.
4. *Old age wellness manager/consultant* We will need specialists to help manage the health and personal needs of an aging population. They will be able to use a range of new emerging medical, drug, prosthetic, mental health, natural and fitness treatments.
5. *Memory augmentation surgeon* Surgeons could add extra memory to people who want to increase their memory and to help those who have been over-exposed to information and need more memory to store it.
6. *'New science' ethicist* As scientific advances speed up in areas like cloning, we may need a new breed of ethicist who understands the science and helps society

---

8. It is, of course not even certain that I will reach 90, even if I avoid accidents.

make choices about what developments to allow. It won't be a question of can we, but should we?[9]

I am fairly certain that the fourth (Old age wellness manager) and sixth ('New science' ethicist) of these jobs will exist in 2025, but whether any of the others will is anyone's guess.

Predicting the future of medicine – an attempt

Let us move on to try to predict the future of medicine. The easy part is predicting the underlying factors that will drive and shape the future of medicine. There is an often understandable human tendency never to be satisfied with what you have or with the current situation, and this will continue to drive medical developments. As long as illness, disease and injury have not disappeared they will be a strong driver for continued medical research. And, as we have become increasingly aware, there is a constant flow of new emerging diseases and new conditions being classified as diseases. Even if we eradicated all illness today, there would be something new to eradicate tomorrow. And even if no more diseases emerged, we would be likely to continue to reclassify previously normal conditions as pathological and in need of medical attention. Such reclassification has social functions and makes it possible for the pharmaceutical industry to offer profitable treatments for the new 'diseases'. An example of this last phenomenon is the classification of social phobias in the most recent version of the International Classification of Disease (ICD 10):

> F40.1 Social phobias Fear of scrutiny by other people leading to avoidance of social situations. More pervasive social phobias are usually associated with low self-esteem and fear of criticism. They may present as a complaint of blushing, hand tremor, nausea, or urgency of micturition, the patient sometimes being convinced that one of these secondary manifestations of their anxiety is the primary problem. Symptoms may progress to panic attacks.

We may all agree that panic attacks do require medical attention and should be classified as a pathological condition, but until recently ordinary 'shyness' would not have been conceived of in this way.

We can also predict that certain social background conditions that shape the future of medicine will remain stable. The most important of these is that the future development of medicine will take place against a background of pervasive inequality both within countries and across the globe. Pervasive inequality has shaped

---

9.   http://sciencesowhat.direct.gov.uk/future-jobs/future-jobs-what-might-you-be-doing.

the introduction of every medical innovation ever made; and given that there is no sign that effective political steps will be taken to remove or reduce inequality, it will continue to shape the medicine of the future. This will entail that even simple and cheap medical treatments will not reach all of those who need them, because not all of those who need them are able to pay. The historical examples are *legio*. Let me just give one. The inactivated tetanus toxoid vaccine, which gives complete protection against tetanus, was invented in 1924. It is cheap to produce and deliver, partly because it does not require refrigeration. Nevertheless, the official WHO/ UNICEF estimate is that only just over 80% of the world population receive this vaccine.[10]

And finally, among the easy factors in prediction we can reliably predict that the path from using a particular medical invention for 'treatment' to using it for 'enhancement' will still be open. This path has been well trodden in the past, and we have no reason to believe that it will not be pursued in the future.

The more difficult part of the prediction, especially in the long term, relates to a set of more variable factors that we can summarise under 4 headings:

1. Which technologies?
2. What conditions?
3. External or internal enhancement?
4. How fast and how far?

■ Which technologies?

We can safely predict that medicine will progress considerably in the next 25 years and immensely in the next 100 years, but it is much more difficult to predict which technologies will be used to treat which conditions.

There is a strong tendency to overestimate the future contributions of any single technology. This overestimation comes about because of two cognitive errors that most of us are prone to. When considering the likely impact of any given technology, say stem cell technology, we tend to forget that there are often several ways of solving a given problem and that even though stem cell technology might solve the problem, some other technology may solve it first or solve it better. Many of the medical problems that stem cell technology might help us overcome have, for instance, previously been identified as the problems that gene therapy would overcome. It is thus likely that any given single technology will eventually only be used to solve a limited range of the problems it could theoretically solve. In ad-

---

10. UNICEF/WHO. Immunization Summary: The 2007 Edition. UNICEF/WHO.

dition, the time it takes for a given technology to move from proof of principle in the laboratory to actual clinical use in humans is often underestimated. We have known for a long time that a Parkinson-like condition in the rat brain can be treated with implantation of dopamine secreting neurons, but we are still some way from making this into a routine clinical treatment in humans (partly because of the large difference in size between rat and human brains). We also tend to forget that many technologies never fulfil their initial promise, or only fulfil it much more slowly than was initially predicted. Many factors may influence technological developments and may lead to a situation where a possible use of a technology is never actually pursued or is quickly given up. As the Concorde and the Tupolev TU144 planes showed, supersonic passenger and cargo flights are technologically possible; but as the demise of both planes also showed, having vastly improved performance (in terms of speed) does not necessarily lead to widespread use.

However, it is nevertheless predictable that stem cell technology, gene therapy and treatments developed on the basis of our rapidly increasing knowledge about the human genome will play a large role in the medicine of the future. Exactly how our genomic knowledge is going to be converted into treatments and preventive interventions is difficult to predict, because the knowledge is likely to influence developments in all of the different branches of medicine. Pharmacogenetic knowledge will, for instance, lead us to use existing drugs differently. But genetic knowledge will also lead to the development of new small molecule pharmaceuticals, like the enzyme blockers currently being developed to specifically target enzymes that are important for specific cancers.

■ What conditions?

What conditions will we be able to cure or prevent in 25 or 100 years' time that we are not able to cure or prevent today?

The scientific developments are likely to lead to new treatments across the whole spectrum of medicine and are likely to radically improve the treatments and preventive interventions for a range of the most common causes of death and ill health. More effective prevention and treatment for ischemic heart disease will undoubtedly be developed, and stem cell treatments will become available for those who nevertheless develop acute myocardial infarction. Many types of cancer will be converted into chronic diseases that can be kept in check (but not cured) by medical treatment. This is already happening for some types of cancer today. In neurology and psychiatry stem cell technology will be used to treat some chronic degenerative disorders, e.g. Parkinson's disease, and electronic man-machine interfacing devices will be used to control a range of other disorders. Vaccines will be developed against many more infectious diseases. Preventive measures will be developed to stop or slow down the age-related decline in muscle strength and bone density. This list could go on indefinitely …

■ What functions will we enhance and how?

It is predictable that many human functions will be enhanced using medical technologies. Treatments developed for muscle wastage in old age or following injury will undoubtedly be used to increase muscle strength (and size) in young adults above what can be achieved by training. And the tendency to use drugs developed for psychiatric conditions as life-style drugs will continue unabated. The prevention of many diseases will also directly lead to increases in function and in average lifespan.

But one interesting question concerns the extent to which future enhancements of function will be directly integrated with the human body. Many bodily enhancements will be integrated, because it is exactly the integration that is wanted. We already have tools that can augment muscle strength far beyond human capacities, but what the bodybuilder or weightlifter want is not the solution to a practical problem of how to lift a certain weight. It is size and muscle strength.

But for other enhancements it is not so obvious that internal enhancement integrated with the body is what will be desired. Let us take cognitive enhancement as an example. It is sometimes predicted that cognitive enhancement will come about either by changes to our brain or by the use of implanted devices. But most people in affluent countries are already massively cognitively enhanced compared to their grandparents, not by having had their brain modified or by having electronic devices implanted and interfaced to their nervous system, but by having access to external enhancing devices. 50 years ago few people could extract the third root of any number without the use of pen and paper, now we can all do it in seconds using a calculator; and due to the internet and smartphones we all have vastly improved and almost immediate access to a wide range of information (and disinformation). This type of external enhancement has several advantages. It does not require surgical intervention so it has none of the risks inherent in surgery; and it is much easier to exchange an obsolete external device than it is to exchange an obsolete internal device. This means that a person will only have reason to pursue internal or integrated cognitive enhancement if it has very significant advantages over the best available external cognitive enhancement. At the moment it is difficult to envisage any kind of internal cognitive enhancement that will have such advantages.

It might be argued that internal cognitive enhancement will come about because we will enhance our children when they are embryos, for instance by the insertion of an artificial chromosome carrying a range of enhancing genes. But even this is

68

a risky strategy, unless the enhancements are very big. The specific artificial chromosome is likely to become obsolete, and it is unpredictable whether any of the enhancements will block further enhancements in the future.

■ How fast will the developments be and how far will they extend?

It is now time for me to nail my flag to the predictive mast and make some concrete predictions for the medium- and long-term future. So here they are. For reasons that have already been discussed, these predictions only relate to the affluent countries; and I am not going to try to predict which countries will be affluent in 25 and 100 years' time.

In 25 years' time medicine will not have changed radically. People will still fall ill, they will still go to the doctor or to hospital, and they will still be treated for their illnesses with surgery and medicines. Treatment possibilities will have been considerably expanded for many diseases, and many cancers will have been converted from acute and life-threatening conditions to chronic conditions requiring life-long management. Preventive medicine will have assumed a greater role, and most people in affluent countries will be taking preventive drugs or having preventive immunisations against common diseases. As a result, the average lifespan will have increased somewhat, but not nearly as much as predicted by Aubrey de Grey, for instance, who claimed in 2004 that "I think the first person to live to 1,000 might be 60 already".[11] Many kinds of enhancement of physical function will have been tried and a few will have become widespread. Cognitive enhancement will still be primarily external, or by small molecule pharmaceuticals.

In 100 years' time medicine will still be around because disease, illness and disability will not have disappeared. Prevention and treatment will still require the input of highly skilled professionals. Whether these professionals will be humans aided by robots and computers, or whether the human doctor will have become superfluous, is an open question. Human bodies will routinely be enhanced, but cognitive enhancement will still be primarily external. The human lifespan will have increased considerably, but will still be far from giving us even intimations of immortality.

---

11. Aubrey de Grey 'We will be able to live to 1,000'. http://news.bbc.co.uk/1/hi/uk/4003063.stm.

Social inequality and 'trickle down' effects

Let us finally return to the issue of social and global inequality in the light of these predictions. If it is true that social inequality is a stable background factor, then we can safely assume that rich and already privileged people and populations will gain access to new treatments and enhancements first. Is this an ethical problem?

Not necessarily. As pointed out to me in discussion many times by H. Tristram Engelhardt, it is close to an analytical truth that somebody must get the new treatments and enhancements first. What is ethically important is not primarily who they are, but what happens next.

If the privileged 1) use their enhancements or better health to benefit the poor and non-privileged, or 2) if the treatments and enhancement 'trickle down' so that over time most or all have access, then the ethical problems are ameliorated. There is little evidence that the rich and privileged have strong desires or willingness to help the poor and non-privileged[12], so here we need to concentrate on the likelihood of the trickle down scenario.

Will new treatments and enhancements trickle down? Trickle down is not an automatic process, as the tetanus vaccination example mentioned above shows. More than 85 years after a cheap technological solution to this particular disease was found, it has still not trickled down to everyone who needs it. We can, however, identify some factors that influence the likelihood of trickle down. A technology is more likely to trickle down if 1) there are big falls in unit price due to mass production (e.g. mobile phones, computers, generic drugs), and if 2) it is of immediate use to the end user (and is therefore likely to be prioritised by the end user). A technology is less likely to trickle down if 1) there are complicated logistics of delivery, 2) it is irreducibly labour intensive at site of delivery, and 3) it is of no immediate use to the end user.

This means that any technology which, for instance, requires surgery to be delivered is unlikely to trickle down effectively unless surgery can be made non-labour intensive. Many kinds of stem cell based therapies or therapies based on implantable devices are therefore likely to remain the preserves of the rich. Trickle down is more likely for small molecule pharmaceuticals as soon as they are out of patent, since their production and logistics can be simplified and their price can

---

12. It might be claimed that cognitive enhancement of some people will in itself lead to benefits for all, since the cognitively enhanced will be able to solve important problems more easily, including problems affecting the poor and powerless. As a conceptual claim this might be true, but whether this will reduce inequality will depend on what problems the increased abilities are directed to solve. There is no *a priori* reason why they should not also in the future be directed primarily towards solving the problems of the rich. The problems of the rich are after all those that it makes most economic sense to solve, because the rich are both willing and able to pay for the solutions.

be kept low. But even here only those technologies that solve problems that are of immediate interest to the end user are likely to trickle down effectively. One of the problems affecting vaccination uptake, for instance, is that although everyone realises its beneficial effects, these effects are not sufficiently immediate to make vaccination a spending priority for someone living at or below subsistence level.

So the final prediction I will make is one I am fairly confident about. The benefits that will flow from medical developments in the next 100 years will not reach everyone who needs them. There will still be large and ethically unjustifiable inequalities in access to good quality medical treatments. As is the case today, only the rich will 'live long and prosper'.

References

Abildgaard, Hanne. 1984-1985. 'Dysmorfismedebatten – En diskussion om sundhed og sygdom i den modernistiske bevægelse omkring første verdenskrig', in *Fund og Forskning*, vol. 27 at http://www.tidsskrift.dk/print.jsp?id=101233.

Byers, John W. 1990. 'Presidential address on the present position and future work of the British Medical Association', in *The British Medical Journal*, Nov 10: 1363-66.

Descartes, René 2010 [1637]. *Discourse on the Method for Reasoning Well and for Seeking Truth in the Sciences*. Translated by Ian Johnston: http://records.viu.ca/~johnstoi/descartes/descartes1.htm.

Tyrrell, David and Michael Fielder. 2002. *Cold Wars: The Fight against the Common Cold*. Oxford: Oxford University Press.

PART II

ETHICAL DILEMMAS

5 Post-What? (And Why Does It Matter?)

Sarah Chan and John Harris

We are all post-simians – but we did not set out to be!

Much has been made recently of the promises and perils of enhancement technologies and their potential to transform us or our descendants into posthumans, beings who are somehow so changed from what we currently regard as human forms and human norms as to be no longer considered the same species or type of creature. Some may aspire deliberately to transhumanity or posthumanity as a goal in itself, often through seemingly far-fetched technological imaginings that include expanding our sensory and cognitive capacities to realms previously unexplored by human beings; extending our lifespans far beyond their current limits, perhaps even indefinitely; achieving new physical feats or powers that are presently outside human capabilities; and so forth.

This focus on such futuristic technologies, whose realisation is still the stuff of speculative fiction, tends to obscure the more mundane circumstances through which what we might call 'posthumans' are likely to arise: through the continuing evolution, via the intersection of biology and technology, of the present human race.

In this chapter we consider the prospect of posthumanity and the ways in which posthumans might come into being. We argue that while the combination of natural evolution and human enhancement may well one day produce beings who might from our present perspective warrant the title of 'posthuman', this is something to be embraced rather than avoided. The transition from human to posthuman in this gradual fashion would in itself be of little moral significance, might indeed go unnoticed. Furthermore, even if technology does enable more immediate transformation, there will be few moral reasons against its use by individuals seeking to attain a posthuman state for themselves or their children. The potential advent of posthumanity, however, should encourage us to rethink our moral attitudes towards species boundaries and towards other biological species, not just in preparation for the posthuman society that may come, but for the world as it exists today.

Human to posthuman: crossing the species boundary

The posthuman state, in most writings, is essentially defined by its deviation from the human state: Hook, for example, writes that "[a] posthuman would no longer be a human being, having been so significantly altered as to no longer represent the human species" (Hook 2004: 2517). Inherent in this definition is also the assumption that the alterations involved in the transformation to posthumanity will be an improvement upon the present human condition, as illustrated in Bostrom's description of posthumans as "beings with vastly greater capacities than present human beings" (Bostrom 2001: 493). The key feature, however, is the extent of these alterations, placing posthumans outside what we currently understand to be our species.

Critics and skeptics of posthumanism have thus focused either on this defining feature of posthumans, the creation of or transformation into a different species, or on the methods used to achieve this transformation. Technology-specific objections to, for example, genetic enhancement, life extension and cognitive enhancement certainly exist and have been well discussed elsewhere, but it is the objections to the putative species transformation that form the basis of most critiques of posthumanism *per se* and by definition, and reveal certain biases and assumptions about the moral meaning of species that bear closer scrutiny.

By way of illustrating the tenor of these objections, consider Nicholas Agar's words on the prospect of enhancement to the posthuman state: "Radical enhancement threatens to turn us into fundamentally different kinds of beings, so different that we will no longer deserve to be called human. It will make us 'posthuman'" (Agar 2010: 2). This is an inherently value-laden description: why should becoming something other than human be regarded as a threat? Why, for that matter, is being called human an accolade that needs to be 'deserved'?

The language of species exclusion often used in critical discourses over posthumanity sets up a distinction between 'us', meaning the human species *Homo sapiens*, and 'them', meaning all other species, including posthumans and also non-human animals.

Again Agar writes, regarding the pleasures of posthuman experience, that "those pleasures will not be ours" (Agar 2010: 127); Leon Kass, considering the prospect of immortality, writes that it would make us "something other than human", that immortals "would not be like us at all" (Kass 2001); Fukuyama worries about the threat to our "common humanity" posed by the posthuman future (Fukuyama 2002), while Habermas warns that "biotechnology will cause us in some ways to lose our humanity" (Habermas 2003). According to these sorts of arguments, then, a strong reason for avoiding becoming posthuman is the very fact that it will make us into something other than humans; in other words, species transformation is itself something to be avoided. The underlying assumption is that human, *Homo sapiens*, is the best species for us to be; that 'we' (whoever we are) should prize our 'humanity' and strive to retain it. Examining this assumption, however, leads us to two questions: what is valuable about being human, and what is actually wrong with either being or becoming a different species?

Enhancement and (post)-human evolution

Let us deal with the simple case first: the species transformation from human to posthuman that might arise through evolution.

The hyper-technological debate over posthumanism often leaves undiscussed the possibility that that these forms of being are simply a probable future consequence of current trends in human enhancement. The lives of present-day humans are already greatly enhanced, at least some of our capacities 'vastly greater', than those of humans living a few millennia or even a few centuries ago – a process of improvement that has taken place through a combination of natural selection and the application of developing technologies such as agriculture, literacy and modern medicine, to name just a few. There is no reason to suppose that (barring planet-wide catastrophe of some sort, perhaps) this process of 'enhancement evolution' will not continue in a similar fashion into the future, incorporating new technologies as they become available and using them, as we have done throughout history, to improve the welfare of humankind. Nor are there reasons to attempt to prevent this: as we have argued elsewhere, there is nothing particularly special about the human species in its present form, save for the fact that it has survived thus far; this alone does not require us to preserve it unchanged in future – particularly if change may increase our chances of continued survival (Chan and Harris 2006). Indeed, if we are able to direct this change ourselves to greater benefit, we ought to do so.

Of course, few do or could rationally support the proposition that we should preserve the human genome exactly unchanged (indeed, as we have previously pointed out (Chan 2008; Harris 2007: 25), the only way to do this would be immediately to cease all sexual reproduction and implement a strict regime of reproduction by cloning only!). Some writers do however reject, either directly or by implication, the application of 'enhancement evolution' to improve human capacities now or for future generations; in other words, they oppose deliberate intervention in the natural evolutionary process to change its course. Whether because of an irrational aversion to interfering with nature, a belief (unjustified in our view) that we should not attempt to author our own destinies, or other reasons, the arguments surrounding this view are well rehearsed and have been considered and rejected elsewhere (see for example Harris 2007). What is clear is that we do already meddle with human evolution in many ways; we are already the products of enhancement evolution, shaped by technology as well as nature. Direct genetic alteration will simply be another means of doing this, to be employed, like many other technologies, when the benefits are judged to outweigh the risks involved.

We can see that, viewed in this way, the process of posthuman evolution has already begun, is in fact a continuum connecting present-day humans with both our human, early hominid and earlier simian ancestors and our potential human and posthuman descendants. Though we can clearly distinguish *Homo sapiens* of the 21st century from the Australopithecines of a few million years ago, or from modern-day chimpanzees and the common simian ancestor we once shared, we cannot point to the exact point at which prehuman became human, or simian became post-simian. Similarly, posthumanity in evolutionary form, when it arrives, will be just one small and indistinguishable step from pre-posthuman, even if perhaps a giant leap (in some ways at least) from what we currently think of as humankind.

In what particular ways, though, might posthumans be different from humans; and why or how would these be important?

What's so special about being human?

The use of biological species as a moral divider, not only to tell us who we should be but to define who 'we' are, who constitutes the group to whom this 'should' applies, is tenuous for many reasons. One difficulty arises from the species concept itself, which is far from unproblematic and subject to numerous possible definitions, not all of which yield consistent results in determining where species boundaries lie (see for example discussions in Hey 2006; Mayr 1996).

It is at present easy to distinguish members of the species *Homo sapiens* from members of other living species, purely through the evolutionary happenstance that there are (as far as we know) no surviving species or subspecies sufficiently closely related to us to cause confusion; for populations of creatures where this is not the case, it is often considerably less easy. We might ask ourselves, if potential posthumans were to come into being, how we would decide whether or not they were in fact human or posthuman. One characteristic often used to determine whether individuals belong to the same species is interfertility, the ability to interbreed. Would we have to subject potential posthumans to enforced reproduction with humans in order to decide whether or not they were one of 'us'?

This speculation, however, while entertaining, ignores the existence of a deeper question, not just how we define ourselves as the human species biologically speaking, but more fundamentally: why does it matter? Attempts to define what is special about being 'human' as opposed to any other species are often phrased in terms of 'human nature' or 'human dignity': Fukuyama, for example, searches for what he calls "Factor X", an "essential human quality" (Fukuyama 2002: 149) that is the foundation of human dignity, "something unique about the human race that entitles every member of the species to a higher moral status than the rest of the natural world" (Fukuyama 2002: 160). Using 'human' as a qualifier both to describe and to circumscribe the group of beings possessing these attributes, however, tends to result in circularity: Factor X not only purports to define what is unique about humans but is defined by its uniqueness *to* human beings. "Factor X cannot be reduced to the possession of moral choice, or reason, or language, or sociability, or sentience, or emotions, or consciousness, or any other quality that has been put forth as a ground for human dignity. It is all these qualities coming together in a human whole that make up factor X" (Fukuyama 2002: 171). In other words, if these qualities were to come together in some other form, they would not serve as the basis for entitlement to the higher moral status supposedly possessed by humans, on the sole grounds that their possessor was not human.

Now, clearly if and while such speciesism holds sway it is better to be human than anything else, non-human or posthuman, but this is like saying it is better to be white in a racist world, or male in a sexist one; it is a reason why under certain circumstances it might be better to choose a particular form of being, not a reason why that form is intrinsically better. To argue on this basis that we should not create posthumans because of how they may be treated is short-sighted; we should instead be arguing for the adoption of a less speciesist view of moral status.

Otherwise, however, it seems that many if not all of the properties that give humans particular moral status, including all the qualities encompassed in Factor X save humanness, are independent of species membership. The use of terms such as 'human dignity' and 'human nature' to denote what is special about humans and, by extension, why we should not risk losing this specialness through posthuman enhancement, is misleading and unjustified (see also discussion in Buchanan 2009). What is special about being human is that humans are a sort of being that generally possesses these valuable attributes, but they are not the only such beings that might do so: posthumans likely will; some existing non-human animals might also; and both should be accorded appropriate moral consideration on this basis, species notwithstanding.

Nicholas Agar has an interesting take on the importance of being human that manages to avoid some of the speciesist pitfalls of accounts attempting to link biological species with moral status. He proposes that being human and remaining so is better *for us* precisely because we *are* human: that as humans, we value "certain experiences and ways of existing" (Agar 2010: 12) that would be lost to us if we were to become posthumans. His account of "species-relative value" does not place humans morally above other creatures; instead it aims to provide a subjective – a species-relative – reason why we as humans should avoid the posthuman transformation for ourselves and for our descendants. While not without its own flaws, this is an intriguing proposition that bears further exploration and that we will return to consider shortly.

Creating posthumans

So far we have considered the potential transition to posthumanism as part of a gradual process – a process, indeed, that is already occurring and may continue to produce, over many generations, beings whom we might consider to be posthuman. But what if this transformation were to happen, rather than by a process of incremental change over a long time, instantaneously or at least within a single lifetime?

There are two ways in which we might imagine applying enhancement technologies to create posthumans: to ourselves, beings currently in existence, or to new beings yet to be created. These two possibilities raise somewhat different issues, though both, we would argue, lead to the conclusion that posthuman enhancement is an acceptable course to chart for ourselves and for our children, should we so desire.

Regarding the prospect of turning existing human beings into posthumans through some technological miracle, we must again ask: why would it be wrong to turn ourselves into a different species? We have argued above that there is nothing essentially preferable or especially good about being human, save for the privileges currently accorded to humans in our anthropocentric world; if the posthuman state offers us opportunities to improve upon current human capacities, expand our experiences and transcend our limitations, what reasons might there be to reject this? This is where Agar's account of species-relative interests and value comes into play, asserting that while there may not be anything intrinsically better about the human condition, we who are currently human stand to lose much of what we value by becoming posthuman.

If this account were to hold true, we would have at least prudential reasons, though not necessarily moral ones, to avoid posthuman enhancement on the grounds that it would deprive us of the experiences we currently value, or at any rate our enjoyment of them. The idea that certain experiences are essentially human and valued by all humans, however, suffers from a number of problems. Do all human beings really share experiences and values that are simultaneously common and unique to humans alone, and is that what makes us a species?

Agar describes these species-relative valuable experiences as "typical of the ways in which humans live and love", "consequences of the psychological commonalities that make humans a single biological species" (Agar 2010: 15). This imputation of biological species from psychological similarity seems to be somewhat backward: surely it is our biological relationship that results in psychological resemblance, not the other way around. If we were to encounter other species with similar psychological tendencies, would we include them on this basis in our biological species? This is hard to imagine. We might, though, recognise them as part of what we might call our moral species – indeed it is to be hoped that we would. Why should we then assume that posthumans will be a different moral species, whether or not we extend to them membership of our biological species?

There is also a difficulty with the assertion that all human beings do share fundamental and essential valued experiences that would be lost were we to become posthuman. Having a sense of value, being able to judge for ourselves what we value, and valuing specific things: all of these are certainly important aspects of human lives. But what it is that we actually value is less species-relative and more individually subjective. For every experience we can think of that an average human might appreciate, we can also imagine a human who might not. Even going beyond superficial preferences (almost all humans like chocolate, but some do not) to the kind of experiences that are supposedly of fundamental value to being human – "the formation of mature interests" and "indefinitely long love affairs" (Agar 2010: 185-6), or (to take further examples from Kass) "natural procreation, human finitude, the human life cycle (with its rhythm of rise and fall), and human erotic longing and striving" (Kass 2003: 20), it becomes ever more clear that not all of us do value these things. The best we could say is that valuing such things might be species-typical, but for an account that relies upon certain shared values being species-definitive, this has little weight.

It may well be true that there is some value in shared experiences, but again, this is a matter of individual judgment and choice as to what value that has, relative to other things we might value. Agar illustrates his views on the value of shared experience with the following example:

> Death and disease present the opportunity for shared experiences ... [T]he sense of belonging that derives from the shared experience has value independent of any useful information. Posthumans permanently immunized against serious disease may provide accurate scientific information about your disease's clinical progression, but they're unlikely to offer insight into what it's like to suffer it. (Agar 2010: 181-2)

The value of shared experience in this guise calls to mind the practice of deliberate HIV infection that exists as a sub-culture within parts of the gay community. To share the experience, not only of the physical disease itself but of the socio-cultural status of being HIV-positive, can be a way of expressing commitment between two individuals, or at a wider level, of belonging to a community – what Dean has described as "experiments with elective kinship" (Dean 2008: 82). This sharing of an experience, despite the danger to health and life it entails, is seen as sufficiently valuable by some to choose this path; others might not agree.

Therefore if, as we have argued, the value we place on experiences, shared or not, is a matter of individual judgment rather than a species-defining property, Agar's argument against posthuman transformation may have some cautionary worth for those who happen to share his values, but it has little moral purchase with those who do not. Alienation from the majority of the human species might be a potential negative consequence of choosing the posthuman path, but some at least seem willing to take that risk (Bostrom 2008).

Posthuman values, enhancement and identity

Another prominent fear in relation to posthuman transformation in the short term is the possibility of losing not (just) our humanity but our individual identity. Kass writes that "a human choice for bodily immortality would suffer from the deep confusion of choosing to have some great good only on the condition of turning into someone else" (Kass 2001). The argument regarding changing values also points to an underlying identity-related problem: if we accept that there are certain things that we currently value (whether species-relative or not), and that we would cease to value as posthumans, and that these things are sufficiently significant to who we are that if we ceased to value them we would no longer be the same persons, then becoming posthuman might indeed turn us into someone else.

Identity-related concerns have been raised in relation to enhancement generally. David DeGrazia, in addressing these, argues that most such concerns stem from confusion between multiple conceptions of identity. He distinguishes numerical identity (whether viewed as a biological or psychological feature) from narrative identity, "what is most central and salient in a given person's self-conception" (DeGrazia 2005: 266), and contends that while interfering with identity in the former sense may be problematic, most enhancement technologies will alter only narrative identity, an alteration which should (if consensual) be acceptable.

Similar conceptual difficulties underlie some of our intuitions about potentially identity-altering posthuman transformations. Agar suggests a thought experiment: what if one could achieve longevity by being turned into a Galapagos tortoise, with an average lifespan of 150 years? He stipulates that patients would "remain conscious … to ensure the preservation of their identities" and speculates that despite this, "few humans would volunteer for the procedure" (Agar 2010: 111). Mere consciousness, however, is not sufficient to maintain narrative identity; the psychological connections between the human state and the tortoise state might be so weak that psychological unity would be destroyed. Becoming a tortoise in this way might constitute an extinguishment of narrative identity such that 'we' would cease meaningfully to exist; alternatively it might simply be a change to narrative identity that most would choose not to pursue. In both these cases we would have good reasons to avoid it. If we are prepared to grant, however, that identity in the sense that it matters to us, narrative identity, can persist even through significant changes in interests, desires and values, then the prospect of these changes alone does not give us a reason to resist posthuman transformation.

Are posthuman values 'ours'? Who are 'we' anyway?

To what extent, then, are our values and interests essential to who we are? The idea that there might be identity-critical values parallels DeGrazia's account (DeGrazia 2005) of possible "inviolable core characteristics" that might be affected by enhancement (an idea that he ultimately rejects on the grounds either that they are not inviolable, or that enhancement will not violate them). It cannot be the case that every interest we have ever held, every passing desire or whim of the moment, is essential to maintaining identity: I may prefer peppermint tea in the morning and Earl Grey in the afternoon, but this does not make me a different person from one time of day to another. Clearly some values are less than fundamental both to humanness and to personal identity. Indeed, through the life course, we are likely to witness significant changes in our own values, desires and interests as part of the natural process of individual human development. Which, if any, of these changes might be identity-compromising – which values are essentially and necessarily 'ours'?

Nick Bostrom presents a dispositional theory of posthuman value according to which posthuman and human values overlap: though our limited human capacities may not allow us to appreciate the worth of certain posthuman experiences, if we were to acquire posthuman capacities, those experiences would be among our values (Bostrom 2001). This analysis is rejected by Agar, who invokes the judgment of a quintessentially human 'ideal self' to deny that the values thus acquired would be 'ours': "humans don't want to listen to posthuman symphonies any more than two-year-olds want to listen to Schoenberg" (Agar 2010: 144).

But the two-year-old may grow up to be an adult who does, in fact, want to listen to Schoenberg; will she then be no longer 'her'? If I have staunchly ignored all music written post-1850 my entire life, then decide at the age of 65 that I want to learn to appreciate Schoenberg and devote time to studying and understanding his music, is this an identity-compromising life choice? Agar does not provide convincing reasons why the process of normal human development from child to adult is to be accepted, along with the radical changes in values and interests it entails, while the process of posthuman development from human adult to post-human, with correspondingly different values and interests, is not. The closest he comes to a justification for this is based in yet another conception of identity: "We invoke a person's long-standing mature interests and commitments in explaining what defines her, what makes her distinctive" (Agar 2010: 186). This may be what defines our identity to others, but it seems unlikely that we have a duty to maintain this externally-imposed distinctiveness, especially in the face of our own desire to develop new and different interests at whatever age.

There is another, deeper problem here in defining what constitutes human versus posthuman values, and hence with the claim that posthuman pleasures 'will not be ours'. The artistic worth of a painting by Miró may not be apparent to an eye unversed in his particular surrealist visual vocabulary, but one can acquire an understanding and consequent appreciation of these artworks without exiting the human species. It is facile to claim that because humans in the past have included Miró's art among their values, it must be among the range of human values and therefore learning to appreciate it does not compromise our humanity. How will we know when the first posthuman symphony is written? If its value is understood only by a composer who appears in all other respects human, the rest of us may think the piece is trash or an "unintelligibly complex racket", but we are unlikely to banish him from the human race merely on account of his poor musical taste.[1] The human will have become posthuman without us realising it.

Acquiring new posthuman faculties, especially by choice, need not compromise our personal identity; nor is our identity intrinsically linked to species or to species-specific properties. Children born deaf can be given cochlear implants to make them hear; this does not affect their numerical identity, and if it does affect narrative identity it does not do so impermissibly – though forcing a deaf person to become hearing against her will might.

Hearing is of course a normal property of the human species, but this should make no difference to the permissibility or the effect on identity of acquiring it. Consider the following example. In subterranean rivers deep within the caves of Mexico, there live certain types of blind, eyeless fish. Acquiring sight would give these fish access to a new spectrum of potentially valuable experiences (allowing, for the purposes of this example, that fish are capable of valuing), in the same way that acquiring UV-vision or sonar could do for humans. One type of eyeless fish, though, is of a species that also includes sighted, surface-dwelling specimens; the eyed and eyeless forms can interbreed freely. Another type is of a separate species,

---

1. In fact on this interpretation, given the propensity of some people to produce "unintelligibly complex rackets", it is highly likely that several posthuman symphonies are already in existence – though (sadly?) unrecognised so far!

all of whose members are blind. If we were to give fish of both species the power of sight, it seems implausible to claim of the second group but not the first that the pleasures of vision would not truly be theirs, merely on the basis that some members of the first species can already see. What if we discovered a tribe of humans with UV-vision? Would we add this to our list of permissible human traits and count the beauty of flowers viewed in the UV spectrum amongst valuable human experiences, or would we call these others posthuman? The species part of species-relativism is unconvincing; and defining what it is to be human by reference to human values, the defining characteristic of which is that they are shared by humans, seems rather circular.

Posthuman children

When it comes to the creation of new beings, the charge of disrupting species-relative values and experiences seems to have even less purchase. The problem of identity rears its head again, albeit in a slightly different form – what we might call the species-identity problem: for whom would it be bad to be one species rather than another? Even if we accept that it might be bad for humans to become posthuman, in the light of the subjective values they currently hold, that says nothing about the objective value of being human versus non-human or posthuman. Going back to the Galapagos tortoise example, if it is not bad to *be* a tortoise, it is not bad to create a being that is a tortoise.

Most of us, though, would probably not choose to have tortoises for children. This points to one reason why we might prefer not to have posthuman children either: we tend to want to relate to our children. Human-tortoise relations may not be as rich and meaningful as human-human relations; it is possible that human-posthuman relations might suffer from the same issue. Agar urges us against enhancing our children to posthuman status for this reason: "We value being connected with our children, even if we know that severing this connection may provide them an objectively superior start in life" (Agar 2010: 191).

This, however, like all the other values we have discussed, is a matter of personal preference. (It is interesting, as a side point, to note that this exact reasoning – the value of sharing experience with children – could also be used to justify deliberately creating deaf children, even though most people would judge being able to hear as an objectively superior state.) It does not show that creating posthuman children (or tortoise children!) would be morally wrong. Nor does it show that it would always be the rational choice to avoid doing so: if we don't see it as important to share experiences with our children, or if we think that posthuman children will still share enough of our experiences to be connected to us, or if we judge that the benefits of being posthuman outweigh the loss of shared experience, then we might be perfectly justified in choosing to have posthuman children rather than human ones.

Our moral species

We have argued in this paper that neither concerns about changing species, nor claims about the objective superiority of being and remaining human, nor worries about loss of identity, nor subjective preferences for certain states of being, provide us with generalisable moral reasons to avoid the posthuman path for ourselves or our children. Becoming posthuman may entail the loss of certain experiences that some humans currently value; these humans will probably choose to remain so, but others who do not share these values might well prefer the posthuman state. Does this, then, leave us hurtling happily towards a posthuman future, and what might we find when we get there?

We noted above that in a world where human beings are privileged over other forms of beings not because of the properties they have but because of a speciesist bias towards humanness as a preferred state, it might be worse to be a posthuman because of the way that beings other than humans are treated. We also noted that this was not a reason to avoid creating posthumans, but an incentive to update our moral maps to something better than the simplistic and speciesist anthropocentric edition currently in common use.

This observation holds a number of lessons, for the human present as well as the posthuman future. First, we should pay more heed to the way humans currently treat non-human beings; second, we should also think not only about how we ought to treat posthumans, but how we would want them to treat others, including humans. Much of the concern about possible posthuman societies centres on the way humans might be treated in a posthuman world, the abuses that might be inflicted upon 'us', the diminution of 'our' rights that might occur once humanity no longer sits unchallenged at the top of the moral hierarchy. On this basis, it might be argued that humans would be wise to refrain from creating the posthuman world, as it would likely be a worse world for them.

We started this paper with the observation that we are all post-simians, but did not set out to be. Given the way non-human primates are now treated by humans, the prudential choice for our simian ancestors, had they been able to exercise it, might well have been to prevent the creation of humans! The fact that we present-day humans are glad that they lacked the power to do so is somewhat irrelevant; if they had been able to make and enforce that choice, we would not be around to be glad. There is certainly no obligation on us to create posthumans just because, once created, they would probably thank us for doing so. Would it, though, be prudential and rational for us as humans to prevent posthumans from coming into existence, for fear of the ways in which they might treat us? Or would it be a better choice for us to try to *be* posthumans? If *someone* will eventually create posthumans, and with them the possibility of posthuman political dystopia envisioned by some, then surely it would be better for us to become posthuman ourselves and at least have the upper hand in the negotiations that might ensue. Even better, though, would be to attempt to avoid such a conflict at the outset. Posthumans would be created by us or from us; in a sense, they would *be* us: our moral species. So far, our moral species is not always very good at recognising members of its own; we tend to get distracted by superficial characteristics such as biological species membership. If we want posthumans to recognise 'us' as belonging to 'them', with all the moral and political rights we wish to retain, we must lay the foundations by developing a moral theory that recognises 'them', along with any other neglected non-human members of our moral species, as belonging to 'us'.

■ References

Agar, Nicholas. 2010. *Humanity's End: Why We Should Reject Radical Enhancement*. Cambridge, Massachusetts: The MIT Press.

Bostrom, Nick. 2001. 'Human Genetic Enhancements: A Transhumanist Perspective', in *Journal of Value Inquiry* 37: 493-506.

Bostrom, Nick. 2008. 'Why I Want to Be a Posthuman When I Grow Up', in *Medical Enhancement and Posthumanity*, Bert Gordijn and Ruth Chadwick (eds). Springer, 107-37.

Buchanan, Allen. 2009. 'Human Nature and Enhancement', in *Bioethics* 23: 141-50.

Chan, Sarah. 2008. 'Humanity 2.0? Enhancement, Evolution and the Possible Futures of Humanity', in *EMBO Rep.* 9 Suppl. 1: 70-4.

Chan, Sarah and John Harris. 2006. 'The Ethics of Gene Therapy', in *Curr. Opin. Mol. Ther.* 8: 377-83.

Dean, Tim. 2008. 'Breeding Culture: Barebacking, Bugchasing, Giftgiving', in *Massachusetts Review* 49: 80-94.

DeGrazia, David. 2005. 'Enhancement Technologies and Human Identity', in *J. Med. Philos* 30: 261-83.

Fukuyama, Francis. 2002. *Our Posthuman Future*. London: Profile Books Ltd.

Habermas, Jurgen. 2003. *The Future of Human Nature*. Cambridge: Polity Press.

Harris, John. 2007. *Enhancing Evolution*. Princeton: Princeton University Press.

Hey, Jody. 2006. 'On the Failure of Modern Species Concepts', in *Trends Ecol. Evol.* 21: 447-50.

Hook, Christopher. 2004. 'Transhumanism and Posthumanism', in *Encyclopaedia of Bioethics*, Stephen G. Post (ed.), 2517-20. New York: Macmillan.

Kass, Leon. 2003. 'Ageless Bodies, Happy Souls: Biotechnology and the Pursuit of Perfection', in *The New Atlantis* Spring: 9-28.

Kass, Leon. 2001. 'L'chaim and Its Limits: Why Not Immortality?', in *First Things* 113: 17-24.

Mayr, Ernest. 1996. 'What Is a Species, and What Is Not?', in *Philosophy of Science* 63: 262-77.

6 Treating Symptoms Rather Than Causes? On "Enhancement" and Social Oppression

Kasper Lippert-Rasmussen

A huge, albeit unproblematic, assumption

Some people's lives are worse than those of others as a result of their being subjected to discrimination. Suppose a couple could prevent their future child being worse off as a result of discrimination by preventing their child from having properties that trigger discrimination. Would they act morally impermissibly if they did so? In this chapter, I defend the view that they do not. However, because my topic raises a number of quite controversial issues, I need to start by saying more about which claims I will not defend, claims which I am not committed to supporting by virtue of my main claim.

Assume that sometime in the future we will be able to, systematically and reliably, change human genes and thereby the phenotypes of future generations. Obviously, this is a huge assumption. But it is also an unproblematic assumption here. First, it is already happening today, though on a rather modest scale, e.g. in connection with the use of pre-implantation genetic diagnosis (PGD) (Green 2007: 2; see also Stock 2003: chp. 6). Second, the issue I discuss here is not whether safe techniques for making genetic enhancements of future generations will ever be available. My issue is this: *If* such techniques are available, should we use them? Affirming the factual antecedent of my question is not necessary to agree with what I say. Accordingly, nor does denying it imply disagreement with me.

Some might motivate a refusal to address my question by complaining that by making the assumption, I am (not by intention, nor by entailment, but *in effect*) giving the false impression that genetic enhancements are feasible and safe, when really they are not. It is like someone discussing the use of nuclear power on the assumption that the technology is perfectly safe, thereby in effect diverting attention away from the real issue: the risks of accidents or nuclear terrorism.

One way to respond to this complaint is to produce a counteracting causal effect. So that is what I will do: I emphatically stress that the reliability and safety of genetic enhancement technologies represent a major issue, and regardless of how the issue I address in my paper is resolved, the issue of possibility and safety remains!

Two kinds of improvement

It is possible to distinguish between two different kinds of genetic enhancements:

Discrimination-independent genetic enhancements, which are genetic interventions that improve the lives of future individuals by means other than ensuring that they do not have properties that tend to result in discriminatory responses that reduce their well-being.[1]

Discrimination-dependent genetic enhancements, which are genetic interventions that improve the lives of future individuals by ensuring that they do not have properties that tend to result in discriminatory responses that reduce their well-being.

Genetic interventions that make future individuals live longer or cause them to be immune to malaria are discrimination-independent genetic enhancements, whereas plausible candidates for pure discrimination-dependent genetic enhancements include genetic interventions that cause people to be heterosexuals.

Many genetic enhancements are really of a mixed type, i.e. they increase people's well-being *partly* because they prevent them from suffering from certain discriminatory responses and *partly* for reasons independent of such responses.[2] For instance, this would be true of genetic interventions that prevent us from developing obesity. Obesity is bad for you because it makes you more likely to develop diabetes and live a shorter, more painful, and therefore worse life. But obesity is also bad for you because you will be less likely to get the job that you have applied for than a person with the right BMI who is no better qualified than you are. Ronald M. Green says this:

Not only do others tend to shun fat people as romantic partners or employees. In addition, they justify these discriminatory attitudes in moral terms. Fat people are seen as responsible for their condition. Research shows that obesity is consistently attributed to laziness and a lack of self-discipline. (Green 2007: 73-74)

---

1. It is common to distinguish between treatments – bringing people up to a relevant species normal standard – and enhancements – raising people above that standard. I use the term "enhancement" (because the term "treatment" would be even more misleading), but not to refer to what this term refers to when it is contrasted with treatment.
2. Relevant here is (Shakespeare 2006). Shakespeare tries to transcend the impasse between the medical model (according to which a disability is an individual bodily dysfunction requiring medical intervention) and the social model of disabilities (according to which a disability is basically a matter of physiologically unconstrained social construction, which bodily conditions count as disabilities).

Discrimination-independent enhancements and my question

I want to set aside the question of what to think about discrimination-independent genetic enhancements. Instead, I focus on what I take to be the harder question of discrimination-dependent enhancements. These two questions are connected, though different.

They are connected because it is possible that some of the reasons that favour or disfavour discrimination-independent genetic enhancements apply to discrimination-dependent enhancements as well. If, for instance, we endorse the former because they improve the well-being of future generations, the very same reason would seem to favour the latter kinds of enhancements.

The two questions are, nevertheless, significantly different, because there seem to be reasons that disfavour enhancements that apply specifically to discrimination-dependent enhancements. One candidate here is the view to which the title of this chapter alludes; in causing future people to not have properties that tend to trigger discrimination, we are really only addressing the symptoms of an underlying pattern of unjust discrimination. Rather than treating the symptoms of allowing the injustice itself to persist, we ought to eliminate the injustice itself. Arguably, no similar objection applies to discrimination-independent enhancements. It is not as if there is an underlying unjust cause of death and that we only treat the symptoms of this injustice if we cause future generations to live for 160 years.

The existence of these specific and additional reasons for opposing discrimination-dependent enhancement makes such enhancements particularly interesting. They represent a harder test case for the moral desirability of genetic enhancements in general. If *even* discrimination-dependent enhancements are morally desirable, then, presumably, so are discrimination-independent enhancements, since any reasons disfavouring these apply to discrimination-dependent enhancements as well, but some reasons disfavouring the latter do not apply to the former.

Double thinking about improving people's lives

Often when the issue is genetic means of enhancement or genetic means of avoiding of disabilities or deficiencies, many people respond by an anxiety-driven kind of double-think. That is, they question whether it really is an improvement of someone's life not to be disabled, not to have reduced learning abilities, or to live longer lives, when these changes result from genetic enhancement. However, the very same people would dismiss with contempt any government official who defends lax safety standards in industry on the grounds that it does not make workers' lives worse, if they become disabled; air-pollution from petrol containing lead that increases the frequency of children with reduced learning abilities on the ground that people's lives are not worse because they experience learning difficulties; or cuts in funding for cancer treatment on the grounds that people are not harmed just because they die at the age of seventy rather than at the age of ninety. And they would dismiss such defences on the grounds that the policies would *obviously* worsen people's lives. Similarly, in their own lives and for their own sakes, they would go to great lengths to avoid becoming disabled and acquiring learning disabilities, and they would definitely not think of the prospect of postponing their time of death 20 years as a "don't care" issue. But all this is double-thinking. If it is worse for you not to have something, then it is better for you to have it. And how the relevant change is brought about is irrelevant to whether it is an improvement of your life.

Genetic interventions – like all other sorts of non-genetic interventions – may make us live better or worse lives. However, fortunately in this paper I can avoid addressing the curious double-thinking just described. My concern is not with improvements of people's lives in general, but with improvements in people's lives that reflect that they are not subjected to discrimination which they would otherwise have been subjected to. So to deny me a topic – to deny that there is anything such as a discrimination-dependent genetic enhancement – you would have to deny that suffering from discrimination in a wide range of cases lowers the well-being of those affected, and that causing people not to posses the relevant discrimination-triggering properties makes their lives go better, all other things being equal. In short, you would not be denying that it is worse to be disabled – you would be denying that it is worse to be discriminated against as a result of disability.

Such propositions tempt no one. If you accept them, you must deny that discrimination makes the lives of the victims of discrimination worse. Hence, you will no longer be able to claim that discrimination is wrong because it harms its victims. But most of us want to say that the fact that Apartheid made the lives of black South Africans worse is at least one reason why it was morally wrong.

Ultimately, we may disagree about what makes our lives go well. The philosophical literature contains competing accounts. One view says that one's life goes better the more pleasant a mental state it contains. Another says that it does so the more of one's self-regarding preferences are satisfied. A third candidate says that one's life goes better depending on the degree to which one realises certain objective excellences. Which of these accounts – if any – is correct is a difficult question. Fortunately, my issue does not require that we settle it. On any of these accounts, discrimination can make one's life worse, whether by reducing the pleasantness of one's mental states, frustrating one's desires, or preventing one's potentials for excelling from being realized.

The goodness of lives: two further specifications

I need to make two further specifications of what I mean by "improving people's lives". First, lives can be evaluated from many perspectives. For instance, we might think Kafka led an excellent life – because he really made something, excellent literature, out of it – while still thinking that many of the rest of us live lives that are much better for us than Kafka's life was for him – because we do not suffer from persistent depressions. When I talk about improving people's lives, I only have in mind what makes people's lives good *for themselves*, not good according to some other standard. The former evaluation is external to the perspective people may have on the quality of their own lives. Hence, discrimination-dependent genetic "enhancements" in relation to hermaphrodites, on my construal, do not imply that the lives of hermaphrodites would be better in this external sense – that hermaphrodites are in any way inferior to other people, e.g. that their interests count for less morally speaking. (That is why I sometimes put "enhancement" in quotation marks.) All I would be implying is that if hermaphrodites were to look at their own lives with an eye to what makes it good for them, they would rightly think that their lives would be better for them had they not been subjected to discrimination because of being hermaphrodites. To quote Jonathan Glover: "To think that a particular disability makes someone's life less good ... does not mean that the person who has it is of any less value, or is less deserving of respect, than anyone else"[3] (Glover 2007: 35).

Second, even if a person is suffering from discrimination that makes her worse off than she would be without it, she might, nevertheless, be worse off without the properties that cause her to be the target of discrimination. So, for instance, homosexuals suffer from various forms of discrimination that they would, on average, be better off without, e.g. hate crimes. But it may also be the case that various aspects of homosexuality make the lives of homosexuals better than the lives of heterosexuals, all things considered, e.g. the experience of being a member of a small and tightly-knit community whose members are self-consciously different. If that were so, genetic interventions to make people heterosexuals would neither qualify as discrimination-dependent nor as discrimination-independent enhancements in my sense, because both of my concepts of genetic enhancement presuppose that discrimination does lower the overall quality of the lives of discriminatees relative to the absence of these properties.

---

3. Obviously, by suggesting that hermaphrodites may suffer from discrimination I do not mean to imply that hermaphrodites are disabled.

My issue: three dimensions

So my issue is the moral desirability of discrimination-based genetic enhancements. But this question can be specified in many different ways. First, we might ask whether we are morally required to perform such enhancements, or whether we are morally permitted, but perhaps not morally required to do so. If parents have an overriding moral duty to make sure that their children have the best life possible, it follows that not having their children enhanced is impermissible for them. However, if other relevant moral concerns are present, e.g. a moral concern for the interests of the parents, they might not have a duty to do so. Few people believe that parents have an overriding moral duty to ensure that their children have the best life possible. In fact, parents may be morally required to sometimes do what is not best for their child, because doing so would harm other children.

Second, there is a difference between asking whether using genetic enhancements is morally permissible (or obligatory) for individual people or couples, i.e. the prospective parents of the future child, and asking whether it is permissible for the group of people consisting of all who may bring into existence new people. The answers to these two questions might diverge, because what an individual couple decides to do has little or no influence on certain patterns of discrimination; whereas what the group of people who bring others into existence do may have decisive influence on whether such discriminatory patterns persist.

Finally, there is a difference between asking whether a couple, morally speaking, ought to perform enhancements and asking whether, morally speaking, it ought to be legal for people to perform such enhancements of their future child (Agar 2004; Bomann-Larsen 2012). The answers to these two questions might diverge because the law solves a collective coordination problem in a way that individual moral duties for parents do not.

My main concern in this paper is to defend the view that it is morally permissible for individual people to have discrimination-based enhancements performed on their future child. In what follows, I want to defend this view against some objections. Along the way, I will say a bit about why I nevertheless think that there might be cases in which the group of people who have offspring are morally required to abstain from such enhancements and cases in which it should, morally speaking, be illegal for individual parents to do what it would be morally permissible for each of them to do (Nozick 1974: 315). Legal moralists – people who think that the law should not forbid morally permissible acts – who accept my core claim about permissibility of enhancement are committed to thinking they should be legal. But as will become apparent, I am not a legal moralist.

Four non-issues: examples, genetic determinism, wrongness of discrimination, and transhumanism

Before I proceed to address my core question, I need to set aside four issues that might blur our focus. First, I have used a few examples to illustrate what I mean by discrimination-dependent genetic enhancements. You might think these illustrations fail. If so, we need not have any quarrel for the purpose of this paper. I am not wedded to any of the examples I have given or will give. All I need to assume is that there are properties such that (i) possessing these properties trigger discrimination; (ii) it harms individuals to be subjected to discrimination on the basis of these properties; and (iii) accordingly, future people will live better lives if, through genetic intervention, we could prevent them from having these properties.

Second, for some, the way I have posed my question may seem to raise the question of genetic determinism, i.e. the view that our phenotypical properties are fully determined by our genes. But in no way am I assuming or believing any such thing. All my discussion presupposes is that genes play a role - not the only role and not even the major role - in determining properties, such as sexuality, that may trigger discrimination. People's heights are affected by their genes, but this does not mean that their nutrition as children or adolescents is irrelevant to how tall they end up being (Lippert-Rasmussen 2010).

Third, the issue I address is not whether discrimination of the sort parents want to shield their offspring from through discrimination-based enhancement is morally wrong. Indeed, I am assuming that it *is* morally wrong. If it was not, discrimination-dependent enhancements would not seem morally different from, say, lifespan-dependent enhancements. The issue is interesting because, arguably, it would be morally wrong to respond to people's unjust treatment of people with discrimination-triggering properties by *accommodating* this unjust response.

Fourth, some people think that there is a morally significant difference between those who want to use gene technology to perfect, or perhaps even transcend, humanity and those who merely want to use gene technology to fight dysfunctions, arguing that only the latter is morally permissible. Along these lines Francis Fukuyama writes as follows:

> And what is that human essence that we might be in danger of losing? ... From a secular perspective, it would have to do with human nature: the species-typical characteristics shared by all human-beings. That is ultimately what is at stake in the biotech revolution. (Fukuyama 2002: 101-2)

This is no insignificant issue, Fukuyama thinks, because morality and human rights are rooted in our shared human nature. Whatever the merits of Fukuyama's worries or other worries about the ambition to perfect humanity, these are not worries that

I need to address for present purposes. Clearly, most people, who are *not* victims of discrimination, are far from perfect and – if you disqualify non-human animals – all of them have "the species-typical characteristics shared by all human-beings". Hence, discrimination-dependent genetic enhancements reflect neither an ambition to perfect, nor to transcend humanity.

Objection 1: Discrimination against existing people

We can now turn our attention to four objections against discrimination-dependent genetic enhancements. The first objection says that there is a moral concern for already existing people who suffer from discrimination because they have the relevant deselected feature. These people are likely to suffer even more if genetic enhancement is used to prevent new people with the relevant feature from coming into existence. Not only does the use of genetic interventions to prevent future people like them from coming into existence send a chilling message to them. As the number of people who deviate from the relevant norm dwindles, it is easy to imagine that their lives will become more difficult in a number of ways. For instance, it might become more difficult to form communities in which they constitute a significant proportion of the population.[4]

Note, first, that this objection at best shows that parents ought to abstain from discrimination-dependent enhancements in some, but not all cases. To see this, let us suppose that up until now everyone has turned out to conform to the relevant norm. However, recently a certain mutation means that, in the future, some people will turn out to be deviant. We also know that these people will suffer various kinds of discriminatory response, but we can prevent any future people from actually suffering such discrimination by preventing any such people from ever coming into existence. If our only objection to discrimination-dependent enhancements is a concern for present people, we would have no reason to reject genetic enhancement in this scenario.[5]

Second, the use of genetic enhancement need not involve any objectionable messages to the people who have the deselected properties. Jonathan Glover puts it this way: "The existence of doctors, hospitals, and pharmaceuticals is not an insult to the sick, just a sign of the platitude that illness impairs human flourishing"

---

4. Objections to preimplantation genetic diagnosis based on the harmful effects on existing individuals or based on the objectionable message that the use of such techniques sends to existing individuals are quite common, e.g. Asch 2003.

5. Similarly, if we could prevent existing, deviant people from being deviant at the same time as we prevented the coming into existence of new deviant people, the present objection would have no quarrel with this intervention.

(Glover 2007: 35). The fact that no one objects to doctors operating on blind people to make them see, but many would object on account of the chilling message sent to geneticists deselecting embryos with genes coding for blindness is yet another sign of the curious double-thinking already in existence. Things might be more complicated with discrimination-eliminating enhancements. Still, I see no reasons why such enhancements, like treatment for blindness, could not be offered in ways that involve no insulting messages.

Third, even in cases, unlike the one I have just imagined, in which a trade-off is present between the interests of future individuals in not suffering discrimination and the interests of already existing people in not being subjected to it, it is not clear that the latter always trumps the former (Savulescu 2001: 423). More generally, imposing costs on existing people for the benefit of future people is not always morally impermissible; for instance, we ought to reduce our emissions of carbon-dioxide to benefit future generations. In sum, while the concern for already existing people points to a relevant consideration, it fails to show that we ought never to implement discrimination-dependent genetic enhancements (Buchanan et al.: 258-303).

Objection 2: To deselect is to discriminate

A different objection says that if prospective parents use genetic interventions to prevent their future child from having a property that tends to trigger discrimination, then in effect they are discriminating against people with the relevant deselected property. Since discrimination is morally wrong, what they do is morally wrong.[6]

In response, I want to defend the following dilemma: either having performed discrimination-dependent genetic enhancements on one's future child does not amount to discrimination, in which case it is not morally wrongful discrimination, or it does amount to discrimination, but then it is not clear that it is always morally wrong to discriminate.

Let me start with the first horn of the dilemma. Consider a couple who use genetic enhancement – in my special sense – to, say, ensure that their child is heterosexual. The parents might be gays themselves who harbour no discriminatory views on homosexuals whatsoever. They simply want their child to live the best life possible and for that reason, and that reason alone, want it to be genetically enhanced in view of the strong and widespread anti-gay sentiment.

Arguably, the case here is really no different from the case of reaction-qualifica-

---

6. For a discussion of this objection, see Dahl 2003.

tions discussed in the discrimination literature (Lippert-Rasmussen 2008). Suppose a bank-owner is totally free from any kind of sexist sentiment. However, she also knows that a lot of her customers harbour such sentiments and that many clients would rather switch to another bank than have a female financial advisor and, accordingly, that she would end up bankrupt if her hiring policy was gender-neutral. So suppose she runs a gender-biased hiring policy solely to avoid bankruptcy. Surely, in one sense of "discrimination", it would seem right to say that, although she treats applicants differently on the basis of sex, *she* does not engage in sex discrimination against applicants, although she takes into account that her customers do. This way of describing the case still leaves it an open question whether she acts in a way that is morally wrong or whether laws should forbid employers from accommodating sexist sentiments in this way.[7] The important point for our purposes is that, similarly, the gay couple described above do not discriminate against gay people even though, in their decision to genetically enhance their child, they accommodate other people's discriminatory responses to gay people.

Admittedly, this is not the only way to describe the situation. Alternatively, we might say that discrimination does not presuppose that the discriminator has any particular prejudice or otherwise objectionable mental states towards the group being discriminated against. After all, there is such a thing as indirect discrimination and, arguably, employers do in a way discriminate against women if they accommodate customers' sexist preferences in their hiring decisions just as a gay couple discriminates against homosexuals if, out of a concern for the well-being of their future child, they use genetic interventions to prevent it from being a homosexual.

In describing the situation this way, we have moved to the second horn of the dilemma, because it is not clear that any differential treatment by an agent that qualifies as discrimination *in this sense* involves this agent's acting in a way that is morally impermissible. Arguably, an employer that accommodates customers' sexist preferences to avoid bankruptcy may not act in a way that is morally wrong and, similarly, nor may a gay couple who discriminate against homosexuals by using genetic intervention to prevent their children from experiencing the same stigma that they have encountered themselves. Saying this in no way commits one to the view that there is nothing morally wrong with the situation. Indeed, what one is saying – given that others *wrongfully discriminate*, it is morally permissible for parents to discriminate in their procreative choices – implies that there is *something* morally wrong with the situation. I conclude that the present argument fails to establish the desired conclusion.

---

7. Recall that the question of morally desirable legal regulation is not my question, viz. pp. 8-10.

Objection 3: We should prevent the discriminatory acts of others

A third objection concedes that people who perform discrimination-dependent enhancements solely for the benefit of their off-spring and on the basis of an unbiased
comparison of the prospects with and without the relevant discrimination-triggering
properties do not themselves discriminate. However, this objection says that, in
taking into account the discriminatory responses of others, people give in to the
unjust dispositions of others. But one ought not to do so. Rather than accommodating many people's immoral tendencies to discriminate, we should change people's
tendencies so that they are not disposed to discriminate.[8]

Note, first, that the last part of this objection seems to presuppose that we have
a choice between accommodating and eliminating discrimination. But, clearly, this
is not the choice faced by the individual couple. Couples can either accommodate
discrimination or have a child that will suffer it. Hence, this part of the objection
fails to show that couples are morally required not to have discrimination-dependent
enhancements performed.

Obviously, the choice situation is different for the group of all couples who have
children, because what they do may make a difference to the persistence of discrimination. To the extent that laws may significantly affect what this group does, it
might even be that the law ought to forbid couples from enhancing their child, even
if it is morally permissible for each couple to do so. One reason why there might
be such a difference is that while the law may change a pattern of discrimination,
the individual couple is powerless to do so.

More generally, if we can collectively eliminate discrimination more easily and
at lower cost than the cost of using discrimination-dependent enhancements to
prevent people who will suffer discrimination from coming into existence, that is
what we should do. However, note that it is not clear that all forms of discrimination can be eliminated easily and at low cost. In effect, we recognize this fact when
we offer cosmetic surgery to people with disfigurements rather than eliminating
discriminatory norms of beauty and looks.

The first part of the present objection points to a slightly different line of
thought; namely that one should not accommodate injustice even though one
cannot eliminate it. Rather, morally speaking, one ought to simply disregard in
one's deliberations the bad effects that follow from ignoring the effects of the
unjust acts of others.

However, it does not seem true in general that whenever people are inclined
to respond in certain wrongful discriminatory ways we should disregard these re-

---

8. Objections of this kind may not have been made in connection with genetic enhancement, but they are quite
   common in relation to other arenas of discrimination, e.g. Wertheimer 1983.

sponses. For instance, suppose that women in mixed prisons suffered from various forms of sexist discrimination and other forms of unjust treatment at the hands of male prisoners. Surely we would not reject the view that, given that we cannot improve the sensibilities of male prisoners to prevent these forms of unjust treatment from taking place, we should separate male and female prisoners to eliminate the opportunity to discriminate on the grounds that this would be giving into the unjust dispositions of male prisoners.

Perhaps there are contexts in which we would say this, but it is not universally true that we should do so. This is not controversial to consequentialists, who think that what determines moral permissibility is the value of the options available to the agent, since these are determined in part by the responses of others, whether just or not. Nor is it controversial for deontologists, according to whom each of us has a special responsibility not to act unjustly, e.g., one has a special responsibility not to discriminate against female prisoners oneself, but no special responsibility for promoting that others do not do so. Hence, like the two previous arguments, the present objection fails to undermine the main claim of this paper.

Objection 4: A concern for our non-discriminatory character

A final argument holds that what makes discrimination-dependent enhancements objectionable is that they imply that we reconcile ourselves to having unjust discriminatory characters, when we should try to improve ourselves. This objection is different from the previous one, because it focuses not on how we respond to the unjust acts of others, but on our characters.[9]

To flesh out this objection, one would have to say more about why we should be concerned with our characters. One view here is that one should be concerned with one's character independently of the acts that it manifests itself in. If that is the reason, we should worry that we are disposed to discriminate against people in ways that we are not aware of, simply because no one has the features that would trigger the relevant discriminatory responses. So if our concern for our character motivates not preventing people from coming into existence who we know would trigger our unjust dispositions, perhaps it also motivates bringing into existence people who might trigger unjust dispositions of which we are presently unaware. Yet, no one, as far as I am aware, favours the idea of broadening the test to which we put our character. But that means they have to explain the moral asymmetry between preventing people from coming into existence who activate discrimina-

---

9. I believe this objection represents the most natural way to develop a virtue ethicist objection to discrimination-eliminating genetic enhancements.

tory responses on the one hand; and refraining from actively bringing people who activate discriminatory responses into existence on the other. This connects with the general discussion of the doctrine of doing and allowing in moral philosophy, which I cannot go into here.

If, alternatively, we should care about our character because of the nature of the acts that it manifests itself in, then it seems that we should be indifferent to our being disposed to act in certain unjust ways, if this disposition will never be activated because no one has or ever will have the features that trigger it. It might be replied that our different dispositions are connected in a certain way and that, by eliminating the presence of one feature that triggers discrimination, we will increase intolerance of the presence of other discrimination-triggering deviations from normality.[10]

Whether this is so is a question of the psychology of prejudice and discrimination. If intolerance of difference works this way, psychologically speaking, there might well be a case against groups of parents, all of whom have one particular kind of discrimination-dependent genetic enhancement performed, since this would simply increase the burdens that bearers of other discrimination-triggering properties would have to bear. But the present consideration would not show that all parents should prevent their children from having any discrimination-triggering properties.[11] Nor does it show that individual parents are not morally permitted to enhance their off-spring, since what one couple does would not increase the burdens on other future people.

Note, finally, that the more one presses the present objection, the stronger reason one has to favour genetic interventions that reduce future people's tendencies to develop personalities involving the tendency to discriminate.[12] Such enhancements qualify as discrimination-dependent genetic enhancements in my sense, although they differ from the ones I have considered so far in that the benefits from genetic intervention do not accrue to those subjected to the intervention but to those whom they would otherwise have subjected to discrimination. Perhaps, while possible in principle, such moral enhancements of human beings will not be on the table for many years to come; but given my initial and, admittedly, huge assumption, this is neither here nor there (Persson and Savulescu 2008).

---

10. For an excellent discussion of the concept of normality, see Glover 2003: 12-13.

11. Again, recall that my topic is what it is permissible for a single couple to do, not what it is permissible for the group consisting of all couples to do, viz. pp. 8-10.

12. I believe an analogous point applies to the first and the third objection.

Conclusion

In this chapter I have discussed four different objections to discrimination-dependent enhancements, arguing that none of them show that it is morally impermissible for individual couples to use such enhancements to ensure that their future child has the best possible life.

I have not shown that there is nothing distinctively objectionable about discrimination-dependent enhancements of people. After all, there might be powerful objections that I have not addressed here. Nor have I have offered any arguments in favour of the view that we ought to make discrimination-independent enhancements of people, partly because the case for making people's lives better in the future speaks for itself (Savulescu 2011; Savulescu and Kahane 2009). Note that, to make my case, I need not even claim that parents have a duty to make their children's lives as good as possible. It would suffice for my argumentative purposes that parents have a duty to avoid harm to their future children when, in the absence of discrimination-dependent enhancements, they would suffer discrimination-related harms. Finally, I have neither argued that it may not in certain cases be impermissible for the group consisting of all future parents to use such techniques, nor that there might not be circumstances under which the state ought to forbid their use.

Still, I have addressed an important challenge to the view that we ought to enhance future generations, and shown why this challenge is much less powerful than sometimes assumed. So, at least, I hope that I have shifted the burden of proof somewhat.

References

Agar, Nicholas. 2004. *Liberal Eugenics: In Defence of Human Enhancement*. Oxford: Blackwell.

Asch, Adrienne. 2003. 'Disability Equality and Prenatal Testing: Contradictory or Compatible?', in *Florida State University Law Review* 35, 318-342.

Bomann-Larsen, Lene. 2012. 'Genetic Enhancement and the Limits to Parental Freedom', in Kasper Lippert-Rasmussen, Mads Rosendahl Thomsen and Jacob Wamberg. Aarhus: Aarhus University Press.

Buchanan, Allen, Dan W. Brock, Norman Daniels and Daniel Wikler. 2000. *From Chance to Choice: Genetics and Justice*. Cambridge: Cambridge University Press.

Dahl, Edgar. 2003. 'Ethical issues in new uses of preimplantation genetic diagnosis: Should parents be allowed to use preimplantation genetic diagnosis to choose the sexual orientation of their children?', in *Human Reproduction* 18.7, pp. 1368-1369.

Fukuyama, Francis. 2002. *Our Posthuman Future: Consequences of the Biotechnology Revolution*. London: Profile Books.

Glover, Jonathan. 2007. *Choosing Children: Genes, Disability, and Design*. Oxford: Oxford University Press.
Green, Ronald Michael. 2007. *Babies by Design*. New Haven: Yale University Press.

Lippert-Rasmussen, Kasper. 2008. 'Reaction Qualifications Revisited', in *Social Philosophy and Practice* 35.3, 413-439.

Lippert-Rasmussen, Kasper. 2010. 'Social constructivism about gender', in *Distinktion* 20, 73-92.

Nozick, Robert. 1974. *Anarchy, State, and Utopia*. Oxford: Blackwell.

Persson, Ingmar and Julian Savulescu. 2008. 'The Perils of Cognitive Enhancement and the Urgent Imperative to Enhance the Moral Character of Humanity', in *Journal of Applied Philosophy* 25.3, 162-177.

Savulescu, Julian. 2001. 'Procreative Beneficence: Why We Should Select the Best Children', *Bioethics* 15.5-6, 413-426.

Shakespeare, Tom. 2006. *Disability Rights and Wrongs*. London: Routledge.

Stock, Gregory. 2003. *Redesigning Humans: Choosing Our Genes, Changing Our Future*. Boston: Mariner Books.

Wertheimer, Alan. 1983. 'Jobs, Qualifications, and Preferences', in *Ethics* 94.1, 99-112.

7 A Liberal View on Liberal Enhancement

Lene Bomann-Larsen

One rough test of whether you regard a justification as sufficient is whether you would accept that justification if you were in another person's position. (Scanlon 2007: 653)[1]

Introduction

Should parents be allowed to design, modify or select genes for the purpose of improving the traits and endowments of their children? Liberal answers vary from the very liberal to the more restrictive. The liberal question of enhancement concerns which procreative measures the state may legitimately permit or prohibit citizens to take by means of law.[2] From a liberal point of view, the baseline is that procreative decisions belong to the private sphere and should therefore be left to parents. Alternative legal principles may seem illegitimately authoritarian, because it appears that the state has no right to interfere with the reproductive choices of citizens.[3]

One liberal reason to restrict parental freedom which has not received much attention, is the claim that children are future citizens – political persons with entitlements – whom the state is obligated to respect. The foundation of my argument is similar to Matthew Clayton's proposal that the ideal of public reason should constrain parental conduct. "Parents should (...) treat their children in accordance with norms that are capable of acceptance by any free and equal person" (Clayton 2006: 92).

The entitlements of future citizens place constraints on what current citizens may permissibly do to them, constraints beyond a right not to be harmed. I suggest they

---

1. Similarly, I would like to invite the reader to keep the following thought in mind: *"What would I accept that my parents did to me?"*, rather than: *"What do I think I should do to my children?"*.
2. In this paper, enhancement should be read as the modification, not selection, of traits.
3. "Prospective parents may ask genetic engineers to introduce into their embryos combinations of genes that correspond with their particular conception of the good life" (Agar 2004: 6).

also go beyond what is ordinarily believed to be violations of the child's "right to an open future" (Feinberg 1994; Buchanan et al. 2000). In the latter view autonomy is understood as an *end-state*, and enhancement will arguably be permissible if it does not narrow, or if it broadens, the range of future life choices available to the child.

Based on the view I expound here, autonomy is a *precondition* of being treated in a certain way. As such, respect for autonomy involves two constraints: there are things one cannot do to others without their consent, and: "Others are not permitted to seek to impart comprehensive convictions to individuals prior to their possession of a capacity for a conception of the good" (Clayton 2006: 103).

As I understand the "precondition view" of autonomy, it is primarily about respecting the other as sovereign, rather than just ensuring that the other becomes an autonomous person (although the latter is arguably an important dimension of parenting as well). Though children are not yet autonomous persons, they will eventually become autonomous persons, and are as such comparable with people who are temporarily incapable of exercising their autonomy. Temporary incapacity does not entail that we can do what we want to someone; we must still treat other people as sovereign. In treating the unconscious patient, the doctor must be able to justify to the person what she does to her. As with all conformity with the requirements of public reason, actual acceptance is not a requirement, but *acceptability* is essential.

The "precondition view" on autonomy is constitutive of legitimate relations between political persons, and has implications for the permissibility of enhancement. Importantly, it implies that enhancement *may* wrong future citizens even when carried out in order to *benefit* them (and even though it actually does benefit them).

The Argument from Extension

It is a problem for sceptics of genetic enhancement that their arguments seem easily fended off with reference to ordinary parental practice: there is simply no reason to think that there is anything peculiar about interventions into the genome that cannot just as plausibly be pinned onto the environmental choices that parents make for their children. Call this *the Argument from Extension*, as it extends ordinary parental practice to cover technological options that are purportedly not relevantly different from non-technological ones. The Argument from Extension has both moral and legal-political implications. If there is nothing special about genetic choices, then as far as morality is concerned what is relevant is whether choices are good or bad, not whether they are genetic or environmental. With regard to legal-political aspects, both the restrictions and the permissions that apply to environmental choices may also apply to genetic choices, when plausible, and likewise with the permissions.

A few remarks: the strength of the Argument from Extension rests on the precise relation between genes and environments in determining phenotypes. Insofar as genes do not strongly determine phenotypical traits and do need "environmental triggers", genetic choices do not appear more invasive than environmental choices. However, in many cases, if the genetic disposition is lacking, it is unlikely that environmental choices alone can make much difference. In that respect, even if strong genetic determinism is false, genes may sometimes matter decisively. And if they didn't – what would be the point of genetic intervention?

Genetic determinism notwithstanding, my concern is the right of parents to *take action* to shape their future children, not the empirical question of whether they will succeed. Of course it is possible to make a genetic choice and not back it up by environmental choices, and hence genetic choices need not give any particular phenotypical results; but it is implausible that parents should go to such lengths as to modify the genetic structure of their children and not follow up by environmental choices; environmental choices which in turn could be futile if the right genetic disposition is not in place. This implies that genetic choices are not identical to environmental choices in terms of the scope of influence these options give parents over their child's development.

The Argument from Extension does not imply that all forms of parenting are morally acceptable. It claims that *even if* many parental choices may wrong the child, for instance by imposing the parents' preferences on the child, we do not and should not for that reason restrain parental freedom. And since genetic choices are not relevantly different from environmental choices in this respect, we are compelled to permit the former. So the argument implies that if we accept parental freedom generally, we are forced to accept that it includes making genetic choices for the child when such choices are technologically possible.

If the practice (of parental freedom) is legitimate in the case of (most) parental environmental choices, why should it not be legitimate in the case of (most) parental genetic choices? Parents are currently allowed to adopt relatively severe educational methods aimed at, for example, transforming their children into successful tennis players or into successful law school graduates. Why should they not be allowed to use genetic methods to achieve the same results? (Mameli 2006: 87)

The problem with this argument is that Mameli seems to accept that parents legitimately use severe methods to transform their children according to their own desires. But that is not necessarily the case. And once we question this premise, we see that the extension is not normatively inevitable in either moral or legal-political terms.

We need to ask what is the specifically *liberal* basis for parental freedom. There are various possible replies. Rawls, for instance, in spite of regarding the family as part of the basic structure of society, does not believe that public reason constraints apply directly to it – though they do apply indirectly in the sense that inequalities within the family must be compatible with equality in the public domain (Rawls 1999). They don't apply directly because the family is regarded a *voluntary* association, and respect for people's right to their own conception of the good, which involves their conceptions of family life and child-raising, imposes a limit on legitimate state interference. But if we consider the child as a political person with entitlements, we are reminded that parental freedom is an uneasy compromise between the rights of parents and the rights of children as future citizens. Children's membership in the family is *not voluntary*, hence public reason constraints may apply directly to the parent-child relationship.

Of course this is a problematic view because children are not yet citizens and do not yet have the conceptions of the good that public reason aims to protect. But public reason constraints on how to respect children create certain *justificatory burdens* on parents. The things that parents do to their children and the choices they make on their behalf should not give these children any just cause for complaint when they eventually grow up.

It is clearly not possible to raise a child in a way that bars *all* complaints; and to some extent complaints may be deemed unreasonable in terms of *necessity*. In voicing her complaints against her parents, the child should take into account that parents have no choice but to let their own conceptions of the good guide them, to a certain extent, in the upbringing of children. But acknowledging this does not invalidate reasonable complaints against parents who make choices that go *beyond* the necessary.

An analysis of the basis for parental freedom reveals why the Argument from Extension does not *compel* us to legally permit enhancement. If we grant that many environmental choices are *necessary*, this does not give us a reason to permit genetic choices which are unnecessary. Moreover, the justification for non-interference with most environmental choices – respect for privacy – does not hold in the technological case, where what is at issue is whether we should permit or prohibit certain services/commodities.

Beneficence

It could be argued that even if it is normatively plausible that moral and legal issues concerning enhancement involve different considerations, it would be wrong of the state to prohibit parents from doing what they morally ought to do, which is to do "what they can to give the child a decent chance of a happy life" (Glover). But how this obligation is to be operationalized is subject to dispute. It may be interpreted both in minimalist and in maximalist ways. Consider a maximalist version, the Principle of Procreative Beneficence (PPB), according to which parents have a positive duty to enhance, as one means of fulfilling the moral requirement above:

> If couples (or single reproducers) have decided to have a child, and selection is possible, then they have a significant moral reason to select the child, of the possible children they could have, whose life can be expected, in light of the relevant available information, to go best or at least not worse than any of the others. (Savulescu & Kahane 2008: 1)

The PPB is developed for selection, not modification, but proponents of enhancement may well believe that the same principle holds in the latter case (Elster 2009). According to Savulescu and Kahane, parents have an obligation to select the *most advantaged* child, which is the one they expect would *benefit more from existing* than any of the others. Under a Principle of Beneficial *Enhancement* we compare possible life courses for the same person, whose life will go *better* if the person is subjected to a particular form of enhancement, rather than being left to nature. To "benefit more from existing" means living a life of greater well-being than comparable lives would provide, and "well-being" is interpreted as a plural concept; equivalent, I take it, to a "good life". "Better" is a comparative term which compares two lives in terms of the degree of well-being they generate.

The Principle of Beneficial Enhancement is ambiguous because the concept of well-being is in itself ambiguous. We lack a unified concept of well-being; hence, we lack a standard according to which different life courses can be compared. Roughly, there are three main conceptions of well-being (Savulescu & Kahane 2008: 5-6; Scanlon 2000: 113). First, an experiental or hedonistic conception, according to which well-being is measured from the "inside", as it were; as the quality of life for the person who lives it in terms of pleasurable experiences. A second conception turns on desire satisfaction or preference fulfilment, again, for the person living the life in question. The third conception is substantive; an "objective list" of factors that constitute well-being; according to which certain activities or properties are intrinsically good for the subject, yet independent of them being actually desired by the subject or of any experienced pleasure they induce. Which of these conceptions should one opt to promote?

Savulescu and Kahane maintain that it does not pose a problem that there are multiple conceptions of well-being. However, this pluralism does pose a problem when the Principle of Beneficence is to be operationalised as an action-guiding principle. The PPB tells us that "wellbeing is to be promoted" (the phrase, not the point of view, is from Scanlon 2000: 108), but in the absence of a specification of the content of well-being, it does not give us any guidance with regard to what we are to promote; and consequently which traits are to be enhanced as conducive to well-being. Take the case of Van Gogh. His manic depression led to a life in the creation of great art, which in some conceptions of 'good life' is highly ranked. However, on a more hedonistic conception of well-being, his life might have been "better" if he had had a stable personality and a "sunny temperament". If his parents had had a choice to "switch off" the gene (assuming that this is a realistic picture) disposing for the condition that made Van Gogh a creative artist but which they could plausibly expect could just as well have led to a ruined life, what should they have done? The problem is that in a case of conflict between values, as in the case just discussed, there is no uncontroversial way to settle the matter. The values involved are incommensurable; there is no common currency or higher value which can be appealed to in order to resolve the conflict (Williams 2002). We may make a choice, but the choice is rather a *leap* than a justified all-things-considered determinate decision based on the weighing of reasons – and some value will be lost as a result of the choice.

Does this mean that there is no way to resolve conflicts between values? In some cases, the answer is yes. These are "tragic" cases, where all options are wrongful choices or will lead to bad results. Yet in many cases there is a way to resolve the problem, even if it is true that there will be a loss of value once one value has been prioritised. For instance, it is obvious that we should break a promise to save a drowning child, even if the value of promise-keeping and the value of saving lives are incommensurable (ibid: 74). Now, if we place ourselves in the shoes of Van Gogh's prospective parents facing a genetic choice, there is no such "naturally obvious" way of solving the case, but it is not strictly a tragic case either. It is not that both of the options are *wrong*; rather, they are both in some sense *right*. However, since there are no means of comparison between the values involved, the parents can only consult their own values; their own conception of the good, which after all they must take to be true. Their own conception of the good is therefore not only all the parents have to go by; it is all they in any conceivable moral sense *ought to* go by (the alternative being to choose something that they believe is not good). There is a conflict here, then, between the moral obligation of parents to choose what they believe is best for their child – a choice which must be based on their own conception of the good – and the political liberal requirement of not imposing one's conception of the good on others. Again, in the case of Van Gogh, his parents would know that a disposition for manic depression could lead to a very difficult life, and would have good moral reasons for doing what they could to prevent their child from suffering such hardships; but their choice to intervene would exclude a disposition for creativity and a life in the production of great art, and arguably make his life go "worse" on this particular parameter. Thus the question arises *with what right* present citizens should be allowed – based on their own conception of the good – to make unnecessary choices about the good of future citizens.

I have suggested that we should accept the force of the Argument from Extension, which implies that this is not specifically a problem in relation to beneficence as a principle guiding *genetic* choices, because exactly the same structural problem relates to all parental choices that aim at what is good for the child.[4] In order to single out which choices – of both kinds – are permissible, we need a morally relevant distinction between choices. Given that we are always in a situation of conflict between values and hence face more or less indeterminacy in our moral choices, I suggest that the rightness of our choices depends on whether they are justifiable to those who are subjected to them. With reference to Scanlon (2000), we owe others a justification for choices that affect them, and the justification must be of a kind that others would be unreasonable to reject. This test of rightness (or wrongness, as Scanlon prefers) is arguably vague – "reasonable" being something of a "magic word" – but given the alternative of prioritising one's own substantive and controversial moral view, an approach akin to Scanlon's seems to be the most promising way of dealing with value pluralism on the moral level.

Just cause for complaint

Granted that there is no cut-off point between genetic and environmental choices, there are some environmental choices which, even when made in order to benefit the child, give the child a just cause for complaint. This is arguably also the case with some genetic choices that are guided by the Principle of Beneficence. But not *all* environmental choices give a just cause for complaint, and hence, not *all* genetic choices will either (the necessity factor notwithstanding). I suggest that a just cause for complaint constitutes the demarcation point between morally permissible and impermissible choices, whether environmental or genetic. I further suggest that what makes for a *just* cause for complaint is whether the intervention is neutral with regard to all reasonable conceptions of the good. This should provide us with a vehicle for determining which kinds of genetic interventions may be legitimately permitted and which may not be, also above the medical threshold.

Say a Benefactor enhances a trait – let us call this trait Memory Type-X – in a Beneficiary, based on the belief that possessing Memory Type-X is better for the Beneficiary than not possessing Memory Type-X. The Beneficiary may reasonably complain that the Benefactor unjustifiably assumes, on the basis of the Benefactor's

---

4. Unless genes determine much more than the environment controlled by parents. In that case the analogy is weakened, and the justificatory burden on genetic choices increases.

valuing of Memory Type-X, that the Beneficiary will or should also value Memory Type-X. The fact that the Benefactor has acted upon an assumption on behalf of the Beneficiary without the Beneficiary having a say gives the Beneficiary a reason to complain that the Benefactor has made a choice on her behalf that the Benefactor had no right to make. By acting on her own assumption about what is good for the Beneficiary, the Benefactor fails to respect the Beneficiary as an autonomous person whose consent should be asked before making that kind of choice for her.

The point is that the Benefactor has no right to *act on* an assumption about what the Beneficiary would value; or more precisely, that the Benefactor gives (or takes upon) herself the right to decide, on the basis of *her* value assumptions, what is good for the Beneficiary. This is a form of paternalism. Paternalism has the curious feature that it aims at what is best for beneficiaries, not benefactors, and when successful a paternalistic intervention leaves the beneficiary better off. And still the beneficiary may *justifiably* complain that the benefactor had no right to intervene, and that – though she is not being used as a means to achieve the benefactor's end – she has been used as a means to promote her own well-being. Again, she might not in fact complain, or want to complain – but she has *a* reason to complain, namely that the benefactor has made choices for her that the benefactor had no right to make.

At this point, two objections may arise. First, would not this also rule out treatment below the medical threshold? Could not the Beneficiary complain that the Benefactor, in intervening to prevent or treat a disease in the Beneficiary, is also acting based on unjustified assumptions about the Beneficiary's conception of the good life, based on the Benefactor's own assumptions about this? Second, if the Benefactor does *not* intervene and Memory Type-X occurs simply due to the course of nature, could not the Beneficiary complain that A *should have* intervened to give her Memory Type-Y instead, if Memory Type-Y is integral to the Beneficiary's conception of the good life?

The response to both these objections turns on *reasonableness*. If the intervention takes place below the medical threshold, we would not think that the future person had a *reasonable* complaint. If the Benefactor, say, "switches off" a cancer gene in the Beneficiary, it would be unreasonable of the Beneficiary to complain that the Benefactor had intervened without a right to do so. The Benefactor may plausibly assume that the Beneficiary would consent to this intervention, just as I may plausibly assume that my neighbour, if he has been run over by a car and is unconscious, would consent to being taken to hospital and subjected to surgery. He would be quite unreasonable to complain afterwards. But the picture would look different if I grabbed the opportunity presented by my neighbour being unconscious to alter his mood because I believed he would be better off being a less grumpy person. Medical treatment is to a larger degree neutral between reasonable conceptions of the good, and it does not normally focus on the identity of the person concerned (at least if we leave out certain controversial cases of mental disease and disabilities). So the complaint that the benefactor makes assumptions about the beneficiary that she has no right to make does not generally hold in medical cases. Of course there are exceptions (Jehova's Witnesses and blood transfusions, for instance). If I *know* that my neighbour is a Witness, he could reasonably complain that I set his autonomy aside – but *only if I knew* that he was a Witness.

As a parent, I have a duty to give my small child treatment if she gets cancer. If I fail, she has a just cause for complaint. But what if I think my child is not pretty enough? Should I give her plastic surgery to make her beautiful? Would that not also give her a just cause for complaint? To me there is an obvious distinction here; the exception perhaps being if her looks were so bad that she really suffered under them. The threshold between medical treatment and enhancement is not fixed or clear-cut. But there is a threshold, and the further we push it and the more options we get, the more we need to let own ideals guide us, and the more reason for complaint we give to those who have been subjected to our ideals without having been asked if they share them.

To the second objection: it would be unreasonable of the Beneficiary to complain that the Benefactor had not intervened to give her Memory Type-Y instead of Memory Type-X because the Beneficiary cannot *demand* that the Benefactor should predict that Memory Type-Y is what the Beneficiary wanted. "You should have foreseen" is not an available complaint to the Beneficiary in this case, as it would require of the Benefactor that she made the *correct* assumptions about what the Beneficiary wanted, with the Beneficiary then blaming her for not making the correct assumption. This complaint is unreasonable because it is *unfair;* it allows for too much (bad) luck. If the Benefactor makes a lucky guess she is in the clear; if she makes an unlucky one she is subject to complaint – and there are so many possible guesses.

It is hard to give examples that bring out intuitions in this context because people have very different intuitions. I have elsewhere tried out the example of life prolongation: suppose your parents have prolonged your life and you really don't appreciate life very much – if you would for that or other reasons prefer an ordinary lifespan, you would have to kill yourself. Who has the right to place you in that position? I get the impression that many philosophers would love the prospect of living for 150 years, and they argue that they would complain if their parents failed to prolong their lives if this option was available to them.

What these philosophers object to is that the *grounds for complaint* are identical in both cases. But to make that case they must hold that the failure to enhance amounts to a *wrongful omission* (otherwise the complaint is not justified.) For failure to enhance to be a wrongful omission there must be a positive duty to enhance which is as strong as the duty to provide medical treatment. I suggested that the justification for intervening medically by gene therapy is derived from the uncontroversial duty to provide medical treatment after the child is born. If it were true that failure to enhance is an *omission,* presumably the duty to enhance must similarly be derived from the obligation to benefit the child in upbringing. But given the range of options available for enhancing different traits, there can be *no omissible duty to enhance any one particular trait.* Thus the future person cannot complain that in their choice between enhancing traits X, Y, Z et cetera, the parents have omitted a duty to enhance trait X or Y or Z. In comparison, operationalising the duty to treat disease D is simple, and the child has a justified complaint if the parents fail to do so.

There is a conceivable situation in which the complaint that someone failed to intervene beyond the given medical threshold seems reasonable. If at a time t1 everyone enhanced the intelligence of their children, any child who had not been enhanced could have a reason for complaint. In that scenario, the "you should have foreseen" argument has some bearing. But in such a situation, it seems the medical threshold has been moved upwards, so that "unintelligent" would be perceived as something of a dysfunction akin to a disability. I do not see any problems with accepting this counter-example. The medical threshold is not written in stone; in other words, the treatability of a condition will in part determine whether it counts as a dysfunction. So at t1 we may well find ourselves in a situation where being stupid is on a par with being sick. My question, however, concerns whether there is a justifiable path to t1, given that we are now at t0.

The fact that there is a basis for reasonable complaint against enhancement is most convincing when a trait X comes at the cost of another trait Y. This gives the Beneficiary a reason for complaint because the Beneficiary might – or at least the Benefactor has no right to assume otherwise – have come to value Y more than X, and the choice of X excludes Y. But there are imaginable cases of enhancement where it seems that *more* X only comes at the cost of *less* X, not at the cost of Y. Intelligence, memory and the like seem to be *enablers of all reasonable conceptions of the good rather than expressive of particular conceptions.* Given their generality, improving such capacities need not entail prioritising one or more particular conceptions. If that is correct, enhancing such traits does not give the Beneficiary just cause for complaint on the grounds that the Benefactor has made unjustifiable assumptions about the Beneficiary's specific conception of the good. The enhancement of enabling traits could be said to provide the Beneficiary with *more* X than she would otherwise have had, but if having *more* X does not entail eliminating, or having less, Y, the reason for complaint is not evident.

If there are traits that are really neutral between reasonable conceptions of the good, these may be enhanced without the enhanced person having a just cause for complaint. Permitting parents to enhance such neutral traits does not seem at odds with a form of political liberalism that takes the claims of future citizens as seriously as the claims of current citizens – because it does not violate their entitlement to their own conception of the good by imposing someone else's conception on them.

Concluding remarks

Convergence between reasonable conceptions of the good in terms of enabling traits is conceivable. Whether there really are any traits that are neutral between different reasonable conceptions of the good is partly an empirical question to which I do not have the answer, but I have some concerns:

Is it true that having more rather than less X does not come at the cost of Y? Consider, for instance, that there are different forms of intelligence. Will a particular type of intelligence, if enhanced, exclude or decrease other forms of intelligence or related cognitive capacities? We could imagine that someone with a talent for mathematics lacked the capacity for others forms of intelligence or other kinds of creativity that are cognitively very different from, perhaps incompatible with, a mathematical way of thinking and problem-solving. And increased memory seems to come at the cost of forgetfulness, which can certainly be an advantage in certain situations.[5] While most of us would certainly find it useful to be able to remember phone numbers and names, there are also many things that are best forgotten. Memory is selective and helps us pick out what is important and relevant. Is it possible to enhance the ability to remember, say, what one has read, while retaining a normal functioning memory in other domains?[6] Again, this is an empirical question, but it needs to be answered before we can conclude that memory is a trait that is neutral between conceptions of the good, and hence that memory enhancement does not give a just cause for complaint.

---

5. In the film *Strange Days* the main character has, like Dumbledore in Harry Potter, saved his memories in a pensieve, which allows him to nurture the memories of his ex-girlfriend to such an extent that he is unable to get on with his life. His friend eventually points out to him that memories are "meant to fade away"; they are "made that way for a reason". I owe this point to Jakob Elster.

6. Research on memory indicates that memory is extremely complex, and that there is no such thing as a unified concept of "memory". While this suggests that the very idea of enhancing "memory" *tout court* seems empirically implausible; it also suggests that "enhancing memory" is not self-evidently a good thing (Glannon 2007).

■ References

Agar, N. 2004. *Liberal Eugenics: In Defence of Human Enhancement*. Oxford: Blackwell.

Buchanan, A. et al. 2000. *From Chance to Choice*. Cambridge: Cambridge University Press.

Clayton, M. 2006. *Justice and Legitimacy in Upbringing*. New York: Oxford University Press.

Elster, J. 2009. 'Procreative Beneficence: Cui Bono?', in *Bioethics* 7. DOI: 10.1111/j.1467-8519.2009.01794.x.

Feinberg, J. 1994. *Freedom and Fulfilment*. New Jersey: Princeton University Press.

Glannon, W. ed. 2007. *Defining Right and Wrong in Brain Science. Essential Readings in Neuroethics*. Washington D.C.: Dana Press.

Glover, J. 2006. *Choosing Children*. New York: Oxford University Press.

Mameli, M. 2007. 'Reproductive cloning, genetic engineering and the autonomy of the child: the moral agent and the open future', in *Journal of Medical Ethics*, 33: 87-93. DOI. 10.1136/jme.2006.016634.

Rawls, J. 1999. 'The Idea of Public Reason Revisited', in Freeman, S. (ed.) *John Rawls: Collected Papers*. Cambridge, MA: Harvard University Press, pp. 573-615.

Savulescu, J. and G. Kahane. 2008. 'The Moral Obligation to Create Children with the Best Chance of the Best Life', in *Bioethics*, DOI:11.1111/j.1467-8519.2008.00687.x.

Scanlon, T.M. 2000. *What We Owe To Each Other*. Cambridge MA: Harvard University Press.

Scanlon, T.M. 2007. 'Contractualism and Utilitarianism', in R. Shafer-Landau (ed.) *Ethical Theory: An Anthology*. Oxford: Blackwell; 644-660.

Williams, B. 2002. 'Conflict of Values', in B. Williams *Moral Luck*. Cambridge: Cambridge University Press, 71-82.

PART III

ARTISTIC RESPONSES

8 Three Ways of Change: The New Human in Literature

Mads Rosendahl Thomsen

In recent years the idea of the new human or the posthuman has gained more attention in literary studies, not just in science fiction studies but also in more general studies of literature. In this article I will argue that literature has dealt with different visions of human change in three distinct ways in the past century and a half, focusing on the mind, the society and the body respectively. After introducing the subject's position in literary studies with examples drawn from Mary Shelley and Don DeLillo, I shall argue that Niklas Luhmann's systems theory can help to differentiate between different ideas of human change. I will then show how literature has responded in different ways to various scenarios for thinking of a new human.

Mixed desires

Developments in biotechnology at present make the future of humanity more interesting than ever and in many ways also more frightening and full of risk. The plethora of possible changes of the human condition offered by advances in human-machine interaction and genetic engineering give the label "posthuman" a substance that also influences how older literature can be read. It is a subject that is important not only for life scientists involved in pioneering research, but also for those working in disciplines as diverse as psychology, law and social science and the humanities.

Despite the potential widespread impact of biotechnology, many people prefer to ignore the issue saying, "luckily I'll be dead and gone when all these things will happen". But 'all these things' refers not only to the more fantastic imaginations of the transgression of humanity, but also to incremental improvements in healthcare and developments that may make a few years difference to average life expectancy.

The fact that the general public finds it hard to relate to the complex issues associated with biotechnical potentials and consequences seems to be underlined by the fact that these subjects have been overshadowed in recent public debate by the issue of climate change. Global warming is a significant change for humanity, but it does not challenge the very essence of what it means to be human, which perhaps makes it less threatening in other respects.

Visions of how the future will play out have had and continue to have a strong influence on the present. In the twentieth century the moon landings and the idea of a space age had a very strong influence; and aside from the technological visions, ideas of worldwide revolutions had a strong hold on people's imagination. For some reason people do not spot as many UFOs as they used to. However, the interest in the posthuman could be said to fill a void left by the absence of extraterrestrial forms of intelligent life.

Some would say that the posthuman condition is not just something to be discussed in the future tense, but that it is a concern of the present, as suggested by N. Katherine Hayles's book *How We Became Posthuman*. This only addresses one subset of the phenomenon (cybernetics), although it is acknowledged that there is more to come (Hayles 1999: 281). Others like Ray Kurzweil in *The Singularity is Near* predict a situation in which machines will become more intelligent than human beings and the Singularity will enforce itself. In Kurzweil's view this day is not too far off, as he predicts that 2045 will be the threshold year (Kurzweil 2005: 136).

At the same time there are plenty of people who feel that the world is not changing so quickly or dramatically. Surgery and medicine may have improved in the past 100 years, but essentially we are still fragile and mortal. There are complicated emotions attached to the notion of whether 'we' are in charge of our destinies. We are more in charge thanks to the potential of biotech, but on the other hand this also spurns the feeling of not being in control because technological development has entered a new phase that seriously undermines the idea of a biological human nature that cannot be altered. There are national and international rules and regulations regarding technologies such as cloning, but many have serious and well-founded doubts about whether they will suffice.

However, these rules and regulations do not restrict the world of fiction, and over the years the issue of the posthuman or new human has been taken up by a range of writers who have often produced works that are both fascinating and frightening. In his most recent novel, *Point Omega*, Don DeLillo has one of his mysterious characters wondering about the human condition in a way that contrasts with the usual discourses on the posthuman with their emphasis on more advanced states:

> ... Do we have to be human forever? Consciousness is exhausted. Back now to inorganic matter. This is what we want. We want to be stones in a field. (DeLillo 2010: 52-53)

DeLillo also presents visions of humanity that come close to Kurzweil's idea of the emergence of a higher intelligence, described in a way that is puzzling, fanciful and frightening. These themes are not new to DeLillo, who touched upon them more than a decade earlier in *Underworld*, which essentially is about the Cold War, but at the end the narrator exclaims:

> Is cyberspace a thing within the world or is it the other way around? Which contains the other, and how can you tell for sure? (DeLillo 1997: 826)

Literature and other arts clearly are in no privileged position when it comes to having a say about the future, and some of the fantasies played out in literary science fictions and films may direct our attention away from the real issues facing humanity. But literature is an art form and a medium that is able to combine the presentation of future scenarios with the exploration of likely human emotions through narratives, and through literature we can gain access to the potential thinking of people from other ages and other cultures which may both inspire us and enable us to identify our own blind spots, thereby contributing to a broader understanding of what it is (and could be) to be human. Not least ideas of what constitutes improvement, perfection and normality should be located in a world view that does not isolate the human body and mind, but sees them as part of a social being with a past, present and future.

Mary Shelley's last man and new man

The British author Mary Shelley wrote about both a new human – or man as was sufficient to say in her day and age – and a last human. What her new human looks like is known to all, being one of the most recognizable faces in modern popular culture, which far exceeds the original text of *Frankenstein: Or the Modern Prometheus* from 1818. It is Frankenstein's creation, a monster brought to life by a young scientist who is out of joint with his own age. The nameless monster is gentle at times, having learned about human behavior from observing a family and reading their books. But he is eventually misunderstood by humans, who cannot see behind his appearance and who think that he is attacking a girl when he is actually trying to save her from drowning. However, the creature is also cunning enough to pin the evidence for the murder of Frankenstein's younger brother on the boy's nanny Justine while she is asleep. The monster is not beyond good and evil, but like humanity he contains both sides.

In the end there is no future for this creation in Shelley's universe, but the creation is used as a vehicle to consider the relations of humans with themselves, the world, and those they have created. Having created another being, Frankenstein suddenly finds himself in a position usually reserved for gods, and the creation does not like the way Frankenstein handles this situation. He asks for a female companion, but knows that Frankenstein is not likely to grant him his wishes:

If you consent, neither you nor any other human being shall ever see us again: I will go to the vast wilds of South America. My food is not that of man; I do not destroy the lamb and the kid to glut my appetite; acorns and berries afford me sufficient nourishment. My companion will be of the same nature as myself, and will be content with the same fare. We shall make our bed of dried leaves; the sun will shine on us as on man, and will ripen our food. The picture I present to you is peaceful and human, and you must feel that you could deny it only in the wantonness of power and cruelty. Pitiless as you have been towards me, I now see compassion in your eyes; let me seize the favourable moment, and persuade you to promise what I so ardently desire. (Shelley 2000: 129)

In the end, despite demonstrating consideration and a gentle manner, the posthuman in Shelley's fiction cannot find a place alongside humanity. The rejection of a new species seems very much to be in concordance with the general sentiment today. We value the unity of humanity, or at least the idea of unity. One thing is that this unity is not reflected in politics, where the realist theory of political power often proves itself right in observing the selfish behavior of nations and the distribution of health and wealth among humans. Another thing is the reluctance to think beyond the human species as we know it and consider what it may evolve into.

Indirectly, Shelley furthered this consideration of the missing posthuman with her novel *The Last Man* from 1826. This novel envisions the end of humanity by way of a natural disaster in 2100, in this case an epidemic. Humanity is not transgressed, and the end of man is thought of not as a continuation or evolution, but as an end played out to the desperate words of Lionel Verney, which also reveal a great deal about the construction of human identity:

I form no expectation of alteration for the better; but the monotonous present is intolerable to me. Neither hope nor joy are my pilots – restless despair and fierce desire of change lead me on. I long to grapple with danger, to be excited by fear, to have some task, however slight or voluntary, for each day's fulfillment. (Shelley 1965: 342)

Such reflections on the boredom of living without others can be found nearly two hundred years later in the writings of Michel Houellebecq, revealing how important the social dimension is to humanity. Still, one is tempted to question why even after Darwin consideration of the idea of human evolution has been limited. Perhaps it is because the time frame in our modern historical conception of time for such change has seemed so long.

The human being according to systems theory

There are many different ways of thinking about the posthuman and human evolution. To bring some order to various literary approaches to the new human, scholars have turned to German sociologist Niklas Luhmann's systems theory (Bruce Clarke in *Posthuman Metamorphosis* (2008) and Cary Wolfe in *What is Posthumanism?* (2010), for instance). Luhmann's systems theory is based on the concept of auto-poiesis, developed by the biologists Humberto Maturana and Francesco Varela as a way of defining life. They define an autopoetic system as something that produces the elements of which it consists and that can discern between itself and its environment (Luhmann 1995: 17). This works on many levels. We know, for instance, that our body renews its cells every seven years or so, but we do not doubt that our body is the same. Life is a process organized by systems or organisms, and when the system stops producing its own elements, life stops.

Luhmann tries to take this further. First by claiming that consciousness is a system – one that produces meaning rather than life. This also makes sense from a phenomenological perspective by asserting the existence of consciousness, a phenomenon that is still difficult to explain fully, but whose reality few doubt in spite of the troubles of pinning it down.

With respect to social systems – communication systems that operate with a logic of their own detached from human intention – Luhmann asserts that such systems are empirical and not merely theoretical constructions (Luhmann 1995: 13). His ideas have been affiliated to all kinds of communication media and to what N. Katherine Hayles calls third generation cybernetics, which is based on the idea of self-organized systems (Hayles 1999: 246; Wolfe 2010: xxi). Luhmann's theory also stresses the mutual dependence of the systems. Changes in one system mean a change in the environment of another and the consequent adaptation that this infers.

Three kinds of human change

Based on Luhmann's theory it is possible to identify three ways of thinking about the new human or posthuman, each with a deep resonance in the 20th century and in the literature of the period.

The first kind of change envisioned was in the mold of Nietzsche's ideas of the superman, namely a human whose mindset had been changed, not least in order to do away with ideas of the divinity and duality, embracing the Earth as man's home (Nietzsche 1969: 42). Less radical versions than Nietzsche's vision of a new humanity developing through a change of mindset are played out in the works of Virginia Woolf, Williams Carlos Williams and Louis-Ferdinand Céline among others. These writers are fascinated with the idea of the new human or a change in the character of mankind, but they also remain skeptical about the gains and profound nature of change by emphasizing how complex the sensations of the everyday are, and how the visions of grand changes are challenged by the routines of the everyday.

The second kind of change has had much deeper consequences in history, namely the idea of creating a new human through a change in society. It is not just a matter of individual change as a form of personal liberation, but the change of a population of a whole society through various forms of educational strategies and use of power. The idea of "new man" has been used as a political rhetoric in a number of societies. The New Soviet Man. The New Chinese. The New Jew. The New Negro (Hellbeck 2006; Cheng 2009). All these labels have been used to promote certain strategies for a change in society which eventually would change humans themselves in a profound way, although these changes are very different from those that machines and biotech might bring about. A less aggressive rhetoric was used, for example, in Turkey after Kemal Atatürk's rise to power after The First World War to further a profound change of culture. Similarly, colonization and missionary work have had a deep effect on numerous societies, documented in literature by Chinua Achebe's *Things Fall Apart*, for instance.

Finally, the possibility of changing human biology in ways that could hardly be imagined before now presents itself as both a reality and a new horizon through human-machine interaction: the potential of cloning, advanced medical techniques and changes in human DNA. This subject has also been addressed in literature as the last frontier of human change beyond that promised by changes in mind and society.

Each of these kinds of change is part of our history of thinking about the posthuman, and each scenario has been dealt with in literature either as a prophesy of things to come or as an attempt to better understand what has happened.

Virginia Woolf's new mind and long memory

Virginia Woolf famously said that human character changed around December 1910, and although it is unclear what she meant exactly – was she talking about literature rather than the world – she was not alone in being interested in a possible change in the way that humans perceived the world (Woolf 1967: 321). Avant-garde movements such as Futurism proclaimed the beginning of a new age, and this idea of the new human following the influences of Nietzsche, among others, was also a preamble for the political rhetoric of the new human.

Despite all the radicalism evoked by movements like Futurism, it is sometimes the more subtle contributions that prove the most important and prescient. Woolf is interesting from this perspective. In *Orlando* which is about a man who travels in time and transcends gender (among other things), she writes:

> The sound of the trumpets died away and Orlando stood stark naked. No human being, since the world began, has ever looked more ravishing. His form combined in one the strength of a man and a woman's grace. (Woolf 1998: 132-133)

This theme of transgressing a border like gender is also central to theories relating to cyborgs. For instance, Donna Haraway sees the realm opened by human-machine interactions as one where gender is transfigured (Haraway 2003: 9).

Returning to Woolf's work, most of which does not contain supernatural figures like Orlando, it is possible to see how she struggles with ideas of the new and the connection between humans, their society and their pasts. For a moment in *Jacob's Room* the hubris of the young students seems to bring everything together – connection and newness:

> They were boastful, triumphant; it seemed to both that they had read every book in the world; known every sin, passion and joy. Civilisations stood round them like flowers ready for picking. Ages lapped at their feet like waves fit for sailing. And surveying all this, looming through the fog, the lamplight, the shades of London, the young men decided in favour of Greece. / 'Probably,' said Jacob, 'we are the only people in the world who know what the Greeks meant.' (Woolf 1999: 101-2)

The importance of feeling a coherence of this kind is a sustained interest for Woolf, and is reflected in her many attempts to make her novels multi-perspective in order to break free from the isolation of the subject. And yet true coherence still cannot be found, so the idea of humanity is fragile:

> Hamlet or a Beethoven quartet is the truth about this vast mass that we call the world. But there is no Shakespeare, there is no Beethoven; certainly and emphatically there is no God; we are the words; we are the music; we are the thing itself. (Woolf 1976: 72)

Woolf writes that she sees this when she has a shock. The idea of the new human puts identity at stake, puts the coherence of humankind at stake, but at the same time she finds no answer to the true nature of humans – only the paradox that there is something that looks like an artwork, but not one that we can believe in. That is unless the evolutionary process is such an artwork, which Woolf herself points to when she describes how she connects with thousands of years of ancestors that have provided her with instincts. In such a way, evolution becomes an enchanted process that provides coherence without submitting to the idea of a creator outside of the world, but to processes within the world. However, for some people the processes of nature were not enough.

The New Man as a political project

Early on in the Russian Revolution, Leon Trotsky said that the ultimate purpose of the revolution was to "master first the semiconscious and then the subconscious process in his own organism." Much later, in the last decade of Soviet communism, a pamphlet declared that the country had become the home of "a new and higher type of *Homo sapiens: Homo sovieticus*" (Cheng 2009: 3). Of course propaganda does not reflect real life, but this propaganda does have the ambition of linking political projects with the idea of having insight into the very nature of human beings, as well as planning how to fix the mistakes of evolution.

What has been produced in the aftermath of such projects is a literature of resistance to such big projects, which more often than not shows how such projects fail because the complexity of material existence, humans and their way of living together are too difficult to figure out. The literature often shows that human identity is connected with memory and laments the last human.

This is the case for the Chinese writer Mo Yan, who has written about both the Great Leap Forward and the Cultural Revolution with great respect for the victims of these historical events combined with a subtle way of showing how irrational desires, imagination and the need for some sort of enchantment work as a destabilizing element that eventually prevents grand projects from becoming reality. His tales are realistic and painful, yet they are also optimistic because they show that no political system can ever gain complete control over the complex beings that are humans. Many of Mo Yan's tales center around the natural world and folklore figures. His approach mixes realistic description with dreamy and fantastic scenarios that apparently counter the pietism of the grand projects.

One story, "Soaring", is the bizarre tale of a young woman called Yanyan who seeks refuge in a tree and refuses to come down despite the pleas of her family:

> "Yanyan," Hong Xi shouted, "you're still human, aren't you? If there's an ounce of humanity left in you, you'll come down from there. (Mo Yan 2001: 94)

The story evolves into a discussion of ethics and whether it is legitimate to shoot Yanyan down:

> In your arms, she's your wife, but perched atop a tree, she's some kind of strange bird. (Mo Yan 2001: 95)

Upon which a policeman shoots and kills her. As she is lying on the ground Mo Yan describes two reactions among the spectators. They want to know whether she is dead, and whether she has feathers (Mo Yan 2001: 96).

The era of grand projects and hyperbolic rhetoric seems to be over. Cambodia under the Khmer Rouge regime was one of the last failed and tragic experiments, at least if one believes that there is no such agenda in North Korea today. But tales such as Mo Yan's or George Orwell's *Nineteen Eighty-Four* still serve as warnings about projects and politics that claim to have figured out exactly what a human being is and what it needs.

Cloning and cult

Biotechnology's potential for changing the human condition has found its way into more literature as the technology has developed. Two very different contemporary authors have made rounded novelistic contributions centered on this subject, namely the French author Michel Houellebecq and the British author Kazuo Ishiguro.

Michel Houellebecq wrote an article a few years ago expressing his desire to be cloned. He started out by saying that he despised himself, but that he could identify even less with his son, since he only reflected half of his genetic code. In Houellebecq's novels two works stand out in taking up the issue of posthumanity. In *Les Particules élémentaires* the postscript describes a transformation of the human that was genetic and applied by UNESCO to create the first new human on 27 March 2029 (Houellebecq 2001: 263). This postscript talks about humanity as the first species able to imagine and enact its own transgression. After criticizing contemporary society in no uncertain terms over the course of the novel, the postscript somewhat surprisingly declares that the book is dedicated to the human.

In *La Possibilité d'une île* the narrative goes backward and forward in time between our contemporary Daniel, who has been cloned more than twenty times in succession to create some kind of illusion of immortality. Sitting in little cells, the clones read about the original Daniel and grow more and more confused about their role. Eventually the 25th Daniel decides to leave his cell, a universe so boring and controlled that the descendants no longer want to live in it, and joins the tribe of mortal humans in the wilderness (Houellebecq 2005: 283).

Houellebecq thereby makes a very effective double critique similar to that of the postscript in *Les Particules élémentaires*: we shouldn't be too happy about our world, but things to come may be worse. More than anything else, the book is a celebration of imperfection. That does not mean that humans should not set goals or aim higher, but that – despite the harsh tone of his work – tolerance is something that should be maintained. And what threatens this *status quo* is, among other things, the cult of the young: a thing that Houellebecq's alter ego finds everywhere in what he calls a perpetual genocide on the elderly.

Another interesting aspect of Houellebecq's novel is of course the scenario that a cult-like group would be able to make radical experiments with human beings outside of democratic control. With all kinds of technology becoming more and more accessible, it is hard not to imagine some mad scientist somewhere trying to be a modern Prometheus – this seems even more likely than the UNESCO model of making advances and new opportunities available to more than six, seven or ten billion individuals.

Kazuo Ishiguro's novel *Never Let Me Go* from 2005, which has now also been made into a motion picture, is set in England in the 1990s and describes Kathy H., who lives among a secluded group of people in the countryside. Gradually the reader discovers that this group consists of clones of other people who have been put into the world to deliver spare parts such as kidneys, livers, etc. for their older duplicates. The reader watches in desperation as these subjects adjust to their fate and talk about being brave during the last phase, when their bodies are emptied of vital organs.

Ishiguro's novel is of course dystopic, and while the theme may seem uncommon at first glance to a writer whose fame owes a lot to the cinematic version of *The Remains of the Day*, it is also obvious that the theme of upstairs and downstairs has been given a further existential turn of the screw in *Never Let Me Go*. An unequal world made even more unequal (Ishiguro 2005: 263).

But one could also hope that Ishiguro's tale now is behind the technological curve. It is likely that human donors will not even be needed in the future, because laboratories can grow – or even "print" – organs, providing a future that in certain respects will be much better than literature could imagine just a few years ago. Still, visions of a better future are a scarce commodity at the beginning of the 21st century.

1960s v. 2010s: What happened to the future?

Literature has been and is a great explorer of the potential reactions of humanity to different scenarios, with the advantage that it can address different aspects of human change alongside each other. But the critical function of literature is also one that could be described as being as much as a vice as a virtue. Idyllic scenarios do not make great literature, but what is perhaps more interesting is that there is often a general disregard in cultural media for what the world will become in the long run. The popular and optimistic images of the space age in the 1960s do not have an equivalent today. Instead, our field of vision is filled with images of the problems of climate changes and the perception of biotech and man-machine interaction as developments that dehumanize. The uncanny aspects of the posthuman and of natural disasters seem to comprise the shared visions of the future, even if less bleak futures seem just as realistic.

Can our excitement about and positive attitude toward the future be regained?

One could argue that art and literature, at least sometimes, should try to present visions in which coherence between body, consciousness (and with that the idea of a self) and society is obtainable. Perhaps art's virtue in this respect is its ability to be both cautious and adventurous in its dealings with future scenarios. In any case, given the historically close links between aesthetics, ethics, and imagination, it is likely that literature and art will continue to make visions of the future and give voice to the emotions that we can attach to complex scenarios that take into account the intertwined relations between mind, body and society, and thus continue to help us imagine things before they suddenly arrive unexpectedly in the world for better or for worse.

■ References

Achebe, Chinua. 2009. *Things Fall Apart: Authoritative Text, Contexts and Criticism*. New York: W.W. Norton & Company.

Cheng, Yinghong. 2009. *Creating the "New Man": From Enlightenment Ideals to Socialist Realities*. Honolulu: University of Hawai'i Press.

Clarke, Bruce. 2008. *Posthuman Metamorphosis: Narrative and Systems*. New York: Fordham University Press.

DeLillo, Don. 1997. *Underworld*. New York: Scribner.

DeLillo, Don. 2010. *Point Omega*. New York: Scribner.

Haraway, Donna Jeanne. 2003. *The Haraway Reader*. New York: Routledge.

Hayles, N. Katherine. 1999. *How We Became Posthuman: Virtual Bodies in Cybernetics, Literature, and Informatics*. Chicago: University of Chicago Press.

Hellbeck, Jochen. 2006. *Revolution on my Mind: Writing a Diary under Stalin*. Cambridge, Mass: Harvard University Press.

Houellebecq, Michel. 2000. *The Elementary Particles*. New York: Alfred A. Knopf.

Houellebecq, Michel. 2005. *The Possibility of an Island*. New York: Alfred A. Knopf.

Ishiguro, Kazuo. 1989. *The Remains of the Day*. New York: Alfred A. Knopf.

Ishiguro, Kazuo. 2005. *Never Let Me Go*. New York: Alfred A. Knopf.

Kurzweil, Ray. 2005. *The Singularity is Near: When Humans Transcend Biology*. New York: Viking.

Luhmann, Niklas. 1995. *Social Systems*. Stanford: Stanford University Press.

Mo, Yan. 2001. *Shifu, You'll Do Anything for a Laugh*. New York: Arcade Publishing.

Nietzsche, Friedrich Wilhelm. 1969. *Thus Spoke Zarathustra*. Harmondsworth, England: Penguin.

Orwell, George. 1949. *Nineteen Eighty-Four*. New York: Harcourt Brace.

Shelley, Mary Wollstonecraft. 1965. *The Last Man*. Lincoln: University of Nebraska Press.

Shelley, Mary Wollstonecraft. 2000. *Frankenstein*. Boston: Bedford/St. Martin's.

Wolfe, Cary. 2010. *What is Posthumanism?* Minneapolis: University of Minnesota Press.

Woolf, Virginia. 1967. *Collected Essays*. Vol. 1. New York: Harcourt Brace.

Woolf, Virginia. 1973. *Orlando: A Biography*. New York: Harcourt Brace.

Woolf, Virginia. 1976. *Moments of Being: Unpublished Autobiographical Writings*. New York: Harcourt Brace.

Woolf, Virginia. 1999. *Jacob's Room*. Oxford: Oxford University Press.

9 Artistic Consequences of Technology Insinuating Itself into the Human Body

Gert Balling

The human body is gradually and increasingly merging with an almost invisible technology in the form of microchips and biotechnology, creating a reconfigured or even enhanced Homo sapiens.[1] When we reconfigure the outer world we redefine ourselves and the world we live in, and at the same time we are redefined by the very same world in a dynamic interaction, a world where it becomes increasingly difficult to define the line between entities like man and technology. What happens when we become manifestations of a man-machine compatibility that until recently only existed metaphorically, but now emerges as cyberbodies?

To the world at large, technical development in the form of gene therapy and cloning is what matters; but to the individual, what matters is finding new points of reference that can define the nature of human existence. Several artists focus on this challenge in perspective of the information society while using the computer as an artistic medium. In this article some of the influential artists within the field will be discussed: Nancy Burson and Keith Cottingham (who work in computer manipulation), and "the living work of art 'Stelarc'" (who is physically integrated in a man-machine installation).

The three artists all include the human body in their works and have a very direct approach to the abolition of the difference between natural and artificial, or rather they address the consequences of technology insinuating itself into the human body. The context is the bearing modern technology has on defining the functionality of the human being.[2]

---

1. The concept of "Homo sapiens 2.0" was launched in 2002, when especially Danish scientists and researchers gave their view on developments within their field in relation to the upcoming cyborg perspectives (Balling 2002).
2. The father of cybernetics, Norbert Wiener, and the computer scientist and literary scholar J. David Bolter both talk of *defining technologies* as technologies that are used to explain contexts outside themselves. These technologies do not have to be the most innovative, but are rather connected to the distribution of technology within the more popular realm.

Photography and computer manipulation

Photography has been used as incontrovertible evidence – a mechanical documentation of reality. This is why photography has been used for visas and passports, documentaries and press photos, the prime task of which is to provide evidence of reality. Private pictures have become proof of man's identity, and public images are signs of a common cultural memory with which people are acquainted thanks to technical reproduction and the circulation of information which follows.

In the electronic mass media of today, photography has changed from the analogous to the digital realm. The digitalized picture, in contrast to the analogue photograph, is dissolved into elements (pixels) which can be manipulated individually, thus making it impossible to trace any manipulation.

Because the digital photograph at least potentially abolishes the authenticity of the picture or representation, the increased use of computers in art photography opens up new perspectives on the 'constructed body'. In these cases artists make use of modern technology such as optical analytical instruments to explore the ways in which contemporary technology influences our understanding of man.

Storytelling systems and man-machine metaphors

However, images of man are not only restricted to the artistic realm. The German computer scientist and theologian Anne Foerst came up with the concept of 'Homo narrandus' to describe man as such as a storytelling animal:

> Why? Because we humans create stories to make sense out of the chaos of our raw perceptions and experiences, to explain ideas and abstract concepts and, ultimately, to deal with the incoherence of this world. To be a human is to constantly weave stories. And to be a culture means to be endlessly woven into a tapestry of more stories. We don't see them as stories because we are so fully embedded in them. (Foerst 2000: 1)

One of the patterns in this tapestry is related to the use of a machine metaphor and technological functionality to narrate ourselves – and, following Foerst, to be able to act in systems, we narrate ourselves and our surroundings into them. We are so to speak narrating the compatibility between man and technology that has now moved from a metaphorical to an implementable level.

The metaphorical anthropomorphising of machine and the techno-morphising of man are closely related and always seem to be in alignment with the state of art in technological development. The tendency to apply state-of-the-art technology as a metaphor for the human body and brain has followed us since the beginning of the industrial revolution, and has been a way of explaining what we didn't understand.

We use the construction tools and systems we have developed according to certain logical and mechanical rules.

It is well known that Descartes' and Newton's ideas became manifest in the French humanoid automatons through the concept of mechanisism. In the early age of the mechanical materialism of Enlightenment the android is perfected in a culmination of interplay between handcraft, art and science. The humanoid automaton is a copy of a human being – an android which at certain intervals gives energy to a transmission system that converts energy into a performing organ. This organ does something that is already scheduled based on the principles for the functionality of the machine, even though the mechanical principle is not visible.

When the universe as well as the human body can be described as a clockwork, it is therefore tempting, in the mechanical materialism, through the technology at hand, to expose the 'secrets' behind nature's processes and functions. The android becomes analysable when machine, movement and the human body are related to one another. The instrument mechanic could, based on the idea of the mechanical functioning body in a mechanical functioning universe, analyse the metaphorical compatibility based on an artificial copying of human movements and actions accentuating the marvels of Enlightenment technology.

A wonderful example of this is the instrument mechanic Jacques de Vaucanson, who created the life-size figure of The Flute Player in 1738. With his mechanical flute-playing android and several other machines, he revealed the mechanical functioning of man to a broader audience.

There are countless well-documented examples of this technological teleological understanding of the world. The clock, the steam engine and later the telephone switchboard have represented the human body and brain and made way for an even closer symbiosis between man and machine through the concept of the computer. The transformation from the mechanical to the computational model marks a shift in focus, because the relationship between the organic and the technological is fundamentally altered through information technology and its paradigms. When the computer was introduced in 1940 it was compared to the human brain, and right from the beginning it was based on a model of how the human brain works. It was understood as an assembly of components, with specific neurons or regions performing memory, sensory, control and motor functions – a universal machine (Nielsen et al. 1990: 308). And at the illustrious American university MIT, the legendary artificial intelligence scientist Marvin Minsky later compared the operations of the human brain to that which can be simulated in a computer. In doing so, Minsky postulated that all brain-based processes can be translated into computer programs (Rötzer 1993: 131).

One of the main factors that change the impact of the technological perspective is the fact that biology has changed dramatically over the last 30 years. Formerly,

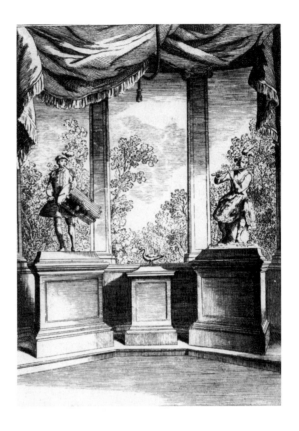

Figure 1. Gravure de H. Gravelot: Frontispice de l'ouvrage de Jacques Vaucanson, *The Flute Player*, 1738. © Musée des arts et métiers-Cnam, Paris / photo P. Faligot.

the domain of biology was focused on the description of species and their origin.[3] However, two events have contributed to a change in this situation: the patenting of life in 1987 with the so called *oncomouse*,[4] and the reported cloning of human embryos in 1993.[5] The biological experiments of the 1980's and the 1990's were directed at optimising man's genetic heritage, and the development within biology relates to the understanding within information science of man as a kind of computer. This is seen, for instance, in Minsky's claim that man can be understood as an information structure. When man is inscribed in the concepts of information theory as a programmable information pattern, man as a unique entity disappears. Jerry Hall, who is a researcher into genes and was head of the Washington University Clinic Laboratory, where human embryos were reportedly cloned in 1993, regarded

---

3. Except for unique cases such as Gregor Mendel's theory of heredity, 1887.
4. In 1987 Harvard University patented oncomouse – a mouse which is genetically predisposed for cancer. Besides general commotion, this patent has led to litigation as to whether life can be patented.
5. In 1993, researchers Jerry Hall and Robert Stillman at the George Washington University Medical School in Washington D.C. carried out an experiment which was reported in the press as the first successful cloning, even though the actual experiment was on artificial twinning using human embryos.

the successful experiments of this laboratory as evidence that it was possible to produce genetically identical copies, e.g. in the form of embryos, which could function as test models, safety copies or stores for spare parts (Bertrand 1994: 125).

The concept of *individual* means literally non-divisible; but in the above-mentioned biotechnological perspective, the idea of man as a unique individual and specimen seems to disappear. Instead it is now the inherited genetic code which is regarded as unique, and thus inviolable. This means that man enters into a relationship of resources as a collection of individual elements or processes. As a resource there is no difference in principle between the technically artificial and the organically natural. In other words, the difference between constructed and living life is abolished. In this perspective, life is not present as a whole in an inviolable individual: life functions according to a more rational logic. So instead of imitating the technological wonders of nature, the nature of man is reformulated according to our technological insights.

The cyborg

The scientific, technical and metaphorical transformation comes to life with the concept of cybernetics, a multi-disciplinary approach with severe cultural and social implications. Cybernetics deals with the organization, control and dynamics of systems, including feedback and interaction processes to obtain balance in such systems, which is also the definition of homeostasis in a human body. Both organisms and machines can be seen as cybernetic systems, and they can both be perceived as information processing systems which are in theory compatible.

The information concept is mathematical and can be measured as a material entity – in bits, which leaves us with the idea of the body as a flow of binary codes and thereby of man as an informational pattern, life as pure information.

The engineer Clynes and the psychiatrist Kline invented the concept of the cybernetic organism, the cyborg, in a paper on a NASA project in 1960. In a more recent interview with Hables Gray, the editor of "The Cyborg Handbook", Clynes recalls the moment:

> I thought it would be good to have a new concept, a concept of persons who can free themselves from the constraints of the environment to the extent that they wished. And I coined this word cyborg. (Gray 1995: 47)

The concept of *cyborg* as a proposal for a new and more flexible version of man for space travel was born: a reconfigured astronaut with machines as natural parts of his or her homeostatic system.

In the perspective of cybernetics, the boundaries of the human can be seen as being constructed rather than given. The flow of information joins the blind man and his cane into one single system – which paves the way for the cyborg of today.

One of the prevailing questions in computer-based or computer-generated cyborg art is whether the nature of Homo sapiens is violated if we can no longer distinguish between animals, humans and technology. A question that itself becomes questionable if we agree that man is actually merging with other information systems, because then the concept of nature as such is no longer an unstable concept. When we as human beings merge physically with other information systems, and they with us, we have a system that is in a state of ongoing becoming through interaction – a complex self-organizing system of multistability.

Burson and Cottingham and the digital merging of man and machine

How do artists like Nancy Burson and Keith Cottingham depict constructed man through modern technology in their most influential artworks? Burson does it by means of the portrait, but not portraits of real people. She works with fictitious people created via a computer-generated fusion of the features of several people. Technically, the tones of the picture have been translated into pixels, after which the computer makes its calculations and "gives birth to" pictures of clones. Burson's series of portraits includes portraits of time-specific types, the so-called First and Second Beauty Composites, where contemporary ideals of beauty are compared with those of the 1950's and with recognisable clones of the power elite with negatively charged titles such as Big Brother or Warhead. Here features of dictators or leaders of the superpowers are recognisable. What is probably her best known picture, the photograph Mankind, shows us the "citizen of the world" – i.e. the computer-generated average human, calculated on the basis of the demographic statistics of the world. Burson's photographs, in other words, are not real portraits but fictitious 'average' people expressed through the form of the portrait.

Burson's portraits do not depict individuals but types. In the typical classical portrait from the Renaissance, the artist depicted certain types with a background setting of external characteristics such as furniture, clothes etc. indicating the person's social rank. Burson, on the other hand, defines the type through the external personal features of the individual as in Big Brother, where dictatorial features are cloned, thus producing a prototype dictator. But does this imply that Burson regards this description of types as being in some way meaningful – in that the exterior of a person reflects features of his character, as the Nazis believed? Or is it all just a post-modern game of quotations, where one is supposed to guess which features are derived from whom?

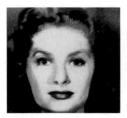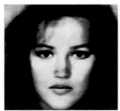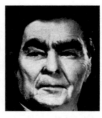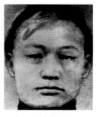

Figure 2-5. Nancy Burson: *First and Second Beauty Composites* (1982), *Warhead 1* (1982), *Mankind* (1983-84). © Nancy Burson/ARKEN Museum of Modern Art. Photo: Planet Foto, Bent Ryberg.

Through the constructions of statistical portraits in computer-manipulated photographs, Burson confronts the myth of the photograph. On the one hand she keeps the categorising function of the photograph, but on the other she distances herself from the photograph as documentation of the reality depicted in it. Burson's statistically calculated portraits draw attention to the photograph as a construct. Digital clones are calculated human beings whose individuality is created on the basis of an individual code at pixel level. In this way, via clear manipulations of the portraits, Burson uses the computer to expose one way of reading man, i.e. as the information structure mentioned above.

The artist Keith Cottingham also takes the portrait as his point of departure. In his series Fictitious Portraits (1992), one sees what looks like a classical arrangement with a half-length portrait of a boy against a black background. The three photographs in the series are called Untitled (Single), Untitled (Double) and Untitled (Triple), showing one, two and three largely identical boys respectively. Cottingham has no real persons as models for these portraits, but has constructed a person on the basis of a combination of himself, drawings, and pictures of different races, ages, sexes, and figures of clay (Cottingham 1996: 160).

These boy figures, then, are fictitious. They are depicted without any individual features: naked in front of a black background. The figures appear with no historical background in an empty space – created by Cottingham himself, who, God-like, has created a prototype which is partly based on figures of clay. A prototype, like Burson's Mankind, that combines the entire world into one creation, here with predominantly Caucasian features. They constitute a unique specimen and are not part of the heterogeneous unity. They each constitute a unity in themselves.

But what are we to call this figure of a boy? What we see is undoubtedly a creature which, looked at from a genetic point of view, resembles a human being. This creature cannot be called a clone, for that would presuppose an original to clone from. Thus it is an artificial, fictitious human being, who both is and is not

134

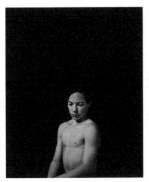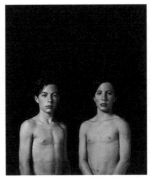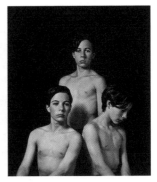

Figure 6-8. Keith Cottingham: *Fictitious Portrait (single)*, 1993, *Fictitious Portrait (double)*, 1993, *Fictitious Portrait (triple)*, 1993. © Keith Cottingham/ARKEN Museum of Modern Art. Courtesy Ronald Feldman Fine Arts, New York / www.feldmangallery.com. Photo: Planet Foto, Bent Ryberg.

a copy of us. Cottingham's prototype is a parallel to us – it is virtually like man, a simulation.

The difference between a person and a simulation is that the person has substance in the shape of a self, which provides a possibility for continuity and individual, human personality. The portrait as we know it from recent times is a documentation of this substance, a documentation of an awareness of consciousness itself – i.e. of what is human.

Here Cottingham stabs rather than pinpoints the function of the portrait. Because the painted or photographed portraits on the drawing-room wall and school photographs placed on sideboards and pianos by grannies, uncles and aunts are documentation. They are memories I can relate to which are exclusively my own. The portrait is my history or the trace of history which creates coherence in an incoherent world. But in Cottingham's boy figure there is no trace of memory or history. The figure is nothing – it is a simulation created on the basis of pixels. If you look more closely at this figure, you will see its lifelessness, its rigidity and the empty expression in its eyes. Has something been lost in translation? Translated he certainly is, digitalised all the way through, and even if he is not derived from an original, he can himself be multiplied. But none of the figures multiplied in the photographs seem to derive much pleasure from this fact.

Nancy Burson's comparison of computer and gene manipulation is a critical contribution to the ongoing debate on gene technology and cloning. Her works are a protest against a view of man in which inherited qualities are seen as decisive for man's character and abilities. This perspective is exposed by Burson as debasing the subject and therefore ethically unacceptable. Keith Cottingham brings into focus digitalisation as a possible, albeit reductive, system for understanding the world.

"Translatable man" is only shown as a simulation of something human, which could be interpreted as follows: if we are made translatable it means that we are no longer human. Both Burson and Cottingham criticise the perception of man as an information pattern as a new absolute.

The Danish biologist Claus Emmeche has sketched the new body perspective in the form of an interface-related perspective where there is less interest in how the body works than in how we can reconfigure the body. The focus therefore changes from how the body works to the extent to which the body can be redesigned and still function (Emmeche 2002: 154). That particular imagination is bound up with our technological and scientific know-how.

The Canadian anthropologist Charles Laughlin follows the tradition of Kline and Clynes on the cybernetic dimension of the cyborg by emphasising a bi-directional penetration process in which the body is physically extended into the world and where the technology is interjected into the body.[6] In this perspective technology becomes part of our perception in an ongoing interchange creating what he calls *cyborg consciousness*. In the process we change ourselves in innumerable feedback processes ending up by "technically transform[ing] our own internal neural processes in order to optimize certain computational abilities [...] that means a process of progressive technological penetration into the body, eventually replacing or augmenting the mental attributes that we normally consider natural to human beings" (Laughlin 1996: 18).

The presentation of the compatibility and the progression of the merge sometimes gives the impression of quite narrow feedback loops leading from wooden legs to replacement or augmentation of structures in the central nervous system, without involving the broad background noise we carry around as members of society and as part of very complex interrelations between nature, culture and other animals.

The American bio- and cyborgologist Donna Haraway made a famous prophecy in the early 90's on rambling dichotomies within the ranks of defining stabilities: Woman-man, human-machine and human-animal (Haraway 1991: chapter 8). But by contrast with Haraway, the present discourse seems no longer to have the perspective of an ironic radical feministic political approach, but is simply a consequence of a technological comprehension of the human body. The metaphorical approach seems in this perspective to be dissolved into images of real reconfigurations and actual enhancements of the body.

---

6. Laughlin's draft on "The Evolution of the Cyborg Consciousness" has been circulated extensively through cyborg-related sites and the like since the end of the 90's. Laughlin has given permission to quote the draft for this text.

Stelarc and the merge of man and machine

In contrast to Burson and Cottingham, Stelarc is his own work of art, in the same way as the artist ORLAN.[7] Nonetheless, he deals with the same questions as Burson and Cottingham. Stelarc has frequently appeared as a performance artist in spectacular stagings, where he is directly plugged into electronic equipment. In his famous performance called Ping Body, Stelarc receives sequences of shocks that make his body perform grotesque patterns of movement. Stelarc has been equipped with a third artificial hand in this performance connected to his own arm by means of electrodes, and is thus automatically directed by the natural movements of his arm, which again are directed by internet actuated and computer-generated electric shocks.[8]

In Ping Body Stelarc stages the body as an information structure: we follow in detail how electric impulses force his body to react in specific ways – as a grotesque updating of Luigi Galvani's scientific experiments with the muscles of frogs' legs and electricity at the end of the 18th century. But he does this in a remotely controlled model, with Stelarc taking Burson's and Cottingham's computer-manipulated body and turning it into reality. Stelarc's scenario of the future is both a modern Gesamtkunstwerk and an electronic horror show. This is partly due to his use of old-fashioned technology in his artistically staged scenarios. Stelarc shows this by means of primitive thick cables which connect him with a control panel, video and computer. Thus the scenario is on the one hand related to the future; but at the same time it is characterized by an aesthetic of decay and disintegration – so-called retro-futurism.[9] In this way Stelarc stages a hopeless image of the future, building on an aesthetics which can be traced back to the laboratories of Fritz Lang's film Metropolis or James Whale's Frankenstein. Stelarc is a freak show, and the audience is both delighted and horrified at the grotesque man-machine apparently deprived of his free will

Stelarc epitomises the cyborg as a concrete expression of man read through the technically oriented conceptual apparatus of information theory as a kind of programmable information pattern and reconfigured man.

Ping Body clearly does not support the myth of man as the controlling subject dominating technology. But still, all the time Stelarc mercilessly manipulates the means in his performance. He is never completely at the mercy of technology, which

---

7. ORLAN transforms cosmetic surgery into performance theatre with herself in the lead.
8. One dimension of Stelarc's performance is made up of sounds created through the stimulation given by sensors on Stelarc's body and his movements.
9. The phenomenon of retro-futurism is prominent e.g. in Ridley Scot's movie Blade Runner, where the visual futurist Syd Mead was in charge of the technical scenario.

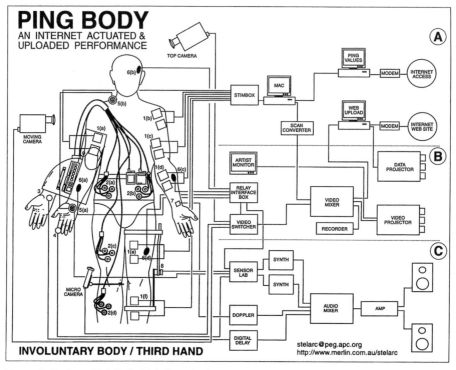

Figure 9. Stelarc: *Pink Body*, Digital Aesthetics, Artspace 1996. An internet actuated & udloaded performance. © Stelarc / billedkunst.dk.

is why technology is also shown as a forceful tool controlled by Stelarc. He stages the shift from the descriptive to a constructive mode by focusing on the development of new technological interfaces between organism and machine – and in that perspective this compatibility must be seen as pointing towards the human being as a machine or machine-compatible system. But Stelarc somehow manages to show that the body is much more than the interaction between body and technology. In the midst of his wild setup – this poetic grotesque – he is a living and experiencing being that feels joy, grief, desire, pain etc., acting out a cultural expression. He is presenting the idea that these qualities, in a complexity perspective, belong to the broad background noise we interact with – beautifully staged in his spectacular circus of Verfremdung.

Outro

There is little doubt that society has evolved at a rapid pace thanks to scientific progress. Today, we live in an information society whose driving force is the production of new scientific knowledge that not only changes the outer world (including interfaces for cyborg reconfigurations of the human body), but also affects the images of man.

Artists challenge our imagination of the technology of tomorrow by presenting scenarios or reflections on implementation scenarios. Where Burson and Cottingham through the cultural history of the portrait raise their voice against genetic reductionism, which in their view debases the subject, Stelarc chooses another path. With his spectacular performances, he shows that he subscribes neither to the fascination with technology nor to technophobia. He shows us an alien world to which we already seem to belong, and which we are therefore forced to reflect upon and act in. He manages to show that when the difference between what is natural and what is artificial is blurred, the values attached to the natural/good and the artificial/bad also disappear.

The cyborg body is neither good nor bad, but serves as an opportunity to reflect upon the stories we weave, such as images of the compatible cyborg.

Parts of this article have previously been published in non-peer-reviewed fora.

■ References

Balling, Gert. ed. 2002. *Homo sapiens 2.0*. Copenhagen: Gad.

Balling, Gert. 2005. *Mennesket er en maskine; Det teknovidenskabeligt kunstigt skabte menneske i et kulturelt imaginært perspektiv* (unpublished PhD dissertation, IT University of Copenhagen).

Bertrand, Ute. 1994. 'Der Entgüldig enfesselte Prometheus', in *Die Geschöpfe des Prometheus – Der Künstlische Mensch von der Antike bis zur gegenwart*, ed. Rudolph Drux. Bielefeld: Kerber Verlag.

Cottingham, Keith. 1996. 'Fictitious Portraits', in Hubertus Ameluxen, *Photography after photography*, eds. Stefan Iglhaut and Florian Rötzer. Dresden: G+B ArtsVerlag der kunst.

Emmeche, Claus. 2002. 'Kroppens kaput som organisme', in *Homo Sapiens 2.0*, ed. Gert Balling. Copenhagen: Gad.

Foerst, Anne. Spring 2000. 'In the Beginning is the Brain (and then comes the Questions)', in *Spirituality and Health; the Soul/Body*. Connection. http://www.spiritualityhealth.com/newsh/items/article/item_55.html.

Gray, Chris Hables. 1995. 'An Interview with Manfred E. Clynes; conducted by Chris Hables Gray', in *The Cyborg Handbook*, eds. Chris Hables Gray, Steven Mentor, Heidi J. Figueroa-Sarriera. New York: Routledge.

Halacy, Daniel Stephen. 1965. *Cyborg: Evolution of the Superman*. New York: Harper and Row.

Haraway, Donna J. 1991. *Simians, Cyborgs and Women; the Reinvention of Nature*. London: Free Association Books.

Laughlin, Charles. 1996. *The Evolution of the Cyborg Consciousness*. http://www.biogeneticstructuralism.com/docs/cyborg_8may96_version2.rtf.

Nielsen, Keld et al. 1991. *Skruen uden ende – Den Vestlige Teknologis Historie*. Copenhagen: Nyt Teknisk Forlag.

Rötzer, Florian. 1993. 'Marvin Minsky; Alles ist mechanisierbar', in *Cyberspace; zum medialen Gesammtkunstwerk*, eds. Florian Rötzer and Peter Weibel. Munich: Klaus Boer Verlag.

Wiener, Norbert. 1948. *Cybernetics: or Control and Communication in the Animal and the Machine*. Paris: Hermann & Cie.

10 Dehumanizing Danto and Fukuyama: Towards a Post-Hegelian Role for Art in Evolution

Jacob Wamberg

Introduction

In his essay on "the new art" from 1925, the Spanish philosopher José Ortega y Gasset famously introduced the notion of "dehumanization" in art (Ortega y Gasset 1948). With this concept Ortega sought to legitimize the abstraction found in contemporary painting: what was encountered inside the frame of art was not to be conceived of as a reflection of the outside – human everyday life – but on the contrary, as a separate aesthetic world devoid of all human and organic traces. In this paper I shall argue that Ortega's idea of "dehumanization" is an early symptom of the posthuman in relation to art, and that the unfolding of the posthuman is therefore not restricted to obvious recent movements such as bio art, digital art or robot art, but should be expanded broadly to so-called modern, or as I prefer to call it, postmodern art as such. According to this reading, the posthuman could be seen quite literally as a qualifying term for the "strangeness" that seems to characterize all postmodern art – modernism invoking posthuman strangeness through abstraction, i.e. the draining of narrative and organic traces from representational images; avant-garde art invoking it rather by intervening with subversive means in the middle of the social sphere.

This posthuman strangeness could also be described as a disjuncture between postmodern art and our inherited art concept – not because this concept is too narrow, but because the very idea of art, autonomous aesthetic expression, appears as the mirror of the inner life of the autonomous human being, so that when the notion of the human becomes strained, so too does the concept of art. This idea I will explore, first, by comparing two exponents of Hegelian evolutionary humanist philosophy: on the one hand the aesthetic Hegelianism proposed by the philosopher of art Arthur C. Danto (1997), and on the other the political Hegelianism and scepticism towards posthuman moves proposed by the political philosopher Francis Fukuyama (2002). Although pursuing quite different kinds of subjects – autonomous artwork and the liberal human being, respectively – both authors put forth evolutionistic chronologies which have reached their absolute end, but in which an attempt is made nonetheless to prolong the subjects' lives by protective measures: art philosophy protecting the autonomous artworks against mere thingness in Danto; humanism protecting the liberal agents against posthuman blunting in Fukuyama.

In my view, Fukuyama and Danto are right in saying that history has reached an end if the subject of history is the liberal human being and its aesthetic expression, art. However, I believe that history could be re-dynamized if we change its subject to evolution as such, i.e. the process of becoming, of assemblages generating new beings. In this expanded scenario the human being emerges not as the end point of history, but rather as a necessary passage through which evolution could reach a new and more complex stage in its continual genesis, a stage that could plausibly be called posthuman. To make such a perspective possible we should, for a start, re-evaluate the nineteenth- and early twentieth-century philosophies of history by Schelling (1978 [1800]), Schopenhauer (1969 [1818]) and Bergson (1911 [1907]), in which nature is in itself an evolutionary project that includes humans and their culture as part of its genesis. In those histories nature's creative forces – the unconscious, will or *élan vital*, respectively – lie beneath and before self-consciousness, the Hegelian spirit, and thus one could assume that the generation of a posthuman stage would comprise a meeting and interlacing of those forces and the products of the human cognitive mind: technology. Here, the experiences of art could turn out to be an important moderator between the forces of nature and technology, as all authors agree that art has privileged access to the subconscious drives of nature. Accordingly, my argument will be that the posthuman qualities of avant-garde and modernist art explore the release of those parts of the subconscious drives of nature that in modern human culture had been imprisoned in the mind and its artistic representations. In the subsequent unfolding of these drives among real things and processes, the drives co-mingle with the products of the cognitive mind, technology, and accordingly trigger a posthuman evolutionary project that comprises both nature and culture.

The Hegelian horizon

If we take my argument at face value, the typical shock reactions that have followed postmodern art whenever it has presented its new methods and materials – from distorted cubist physiognomies to empty galleries, from exploding machines to genetically modified green rabbits – are thus quite sound. Postmodern art is indeed strange because it explores a world that is becoming increasingly alienated from human life as we thought we had come to know it. Ortega (1948: 5) defended this dehumanized world by isolating it to a purely imaginary, aesthetic sphere, separated from the everyday world of the masses, who he thought would never be able to understand it. Yet as I see it, abstract art rather functions as a laboratory for dehumanizing tendencies, which are already interfering in so-called everyday life – a life whose days are, in fact, steadily becoming unlike each other, as accelerating technology makes them increasingly less just-human.

The celebrated duality between 'progressive' avant-garde and 'reactionary' modernism – between on the one hand, a politically ambitious, form-negating, re-circulating and everyday-near art (Bürger 1984 [1980, 1974]) and on the other hand a politically inactive, form-fetichizing, originality-postulating and everyday-alienated modernism (Greenberg 1986 [1939]) – thus does not hold water. As seen through a dehumanized posthuman lens, modernism's many experiments with deformation of the human body and diverse kinds of non-figuration – what Ortega terms for instance the modernist's "startling fauna", the "human aspect which he destroys" (1948: 22) – appear just as radical as their "avant-garde" counterparts: bound to representational media inside frames not because of conservatism but rather because they are posthuman visions which cannot yet be realized in those physical surroundings towards which the avant-gardes typically are oriented. For example, when the female models of the Danish modernist painter Vilhelm Lundstrøm appear without faces, this seems to be not only formalist abstractions with exclusively aesthetic content but rather an investigation of posthuman non-identity – pointing forward to, say, Assiz and Cucher's faceless digital photographs, which are difficult *not* to insert in a posthuman perspective, and thereby too, to the first realization in actual flesh of such visions: ORLAN's remodelling of her own body through artistic actions of plastic surgery.

In addition to such alienation of human flesh forms, postmodern art also appears strange, simply because it seems alienated from the concept of art itself: the idea of autonomous art. This happens in the many avant-garde manifestations in which the artistic activities become so intertwined in diverse reality domains – physical spaces, concepts, situations, mass and digital media, or, as indeed in ORLAN, biological beings – that the specifically artistic dimension seems hard to separate from those realities. The philosopher and art critic Arthur C. Danto has famously sought to solve this problem in an art-genealogical light derived from Hegel, the German idealist philosopher. According to Hegel's lectures on aesthetics, held in Berlin in the 1820s (Hegel 1975 [1835]), at that time art was already approaching its end as a primary medium of human insight, because as history was getting close to its fulfilment, consisting of the world spirit's – the motor of the world – getting to know itself and transparently seeing through the world, only philosophy, pure spiritual knowledge, would be adequate as insight and therefore would outdistance the more matter-bound media of art. According to Danto, the collapse into reality of twentieth-century art phenomena, such as (allegedly) Warhol's Brillo Boxes, represents this Hegelian end of art (Danto 1997; Danto 1986). In these utterly prosaic objects art is already outdistanced by philosophy, its own philosophy, so that the object itself is dead as art and indistinguishable from the rest of the prosaic world. Nevertheless, the object acquires a prolonged, in principle eternal life as art from a protective cloud of philosophy, a dazzle of self-reflectivity, upholding that distinction between art and non-art, which the object itself is too weak to maintain. In Danto's view, then, art is led into a zombie-like double existence, having both outlived itself and been kept eternally alive in the respirator of art philosophy.

Danto's analysis is purely humanist, freezing the history of art into its limbo-like afterlife at the point when human consciousness has recognized what art is and can do. However, Hegelian philosophy of history is pressed more explicitly by posthumanism by another contributor to this anthology, the political philosopher Francis Fukuyama. To be sure, in Fukuyama's breakthrough, *The End of History and the Last Man* (Fukuyama 1992), the political fate of humankind after the crumbling of East Bloc communism was updated according to the 1930s reading of Hegel's

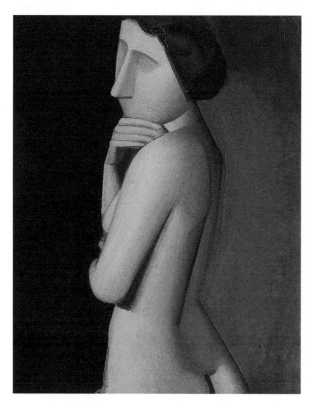

Figure 1. Vilhelm Lundstrøm, *Standing model* (1930-32), oil on canvas. © Malmö Art Museum, Vilhelm Lundstrøm/ Billedkunst.dk.

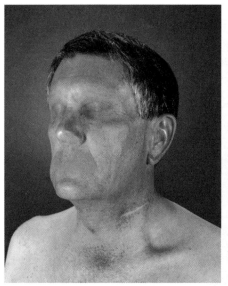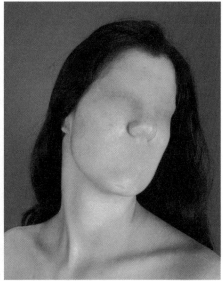

Figure 2 + 3. Assiz and Cucher, *George* and *Maria* (1994), computer-manipulated photographs. © Assiz and Cucher.

Phenomenology of Spirit by Alexandre Kojève, the Russian-French philosopher. In Fukuyama's elegant performance, an attempt is made to demonstrate that the final political horizon of the human being is liberal democracy because this system most adequately fulfils a fundamental desire in humans: the desire for recognition, the Greek *thymos*, by fellow beings. According to Hegel and Kojève's evolutionary narrative, in the ancient beginnings of culture this desire was fulfilled by risking one's own life in battle: the winner gained recognition from the conquered party, who became a slave (Kojève 1969 [1947]). However, as it was unsatisfying in the long run to get recognition from someone beneath you in value, recognition gradually shifted to something obtained by the slave through his sublimating activity, work – first from the new immaterial God for whom everybody was equal in the afterlife, then from the fellow slaves who in the meantime had turned into democratic citizens giving each other recognition through the common societal duty of work. It is this tendency, Fukuyama observes, which spreads universally in the late twentieth century, in which first the Latin American fascist regimes, then the East Bloc communist regimes, allegedly gave way to liberal democracy.

Just as it is impossible in Danto's artistic narrative to envision a future for art after art has been philosophically comprehended, so it is impossible in Fukuyama's political narrative to envision a future for the human being after the fundamental human desire for recognition has been both philosophically comprehended and

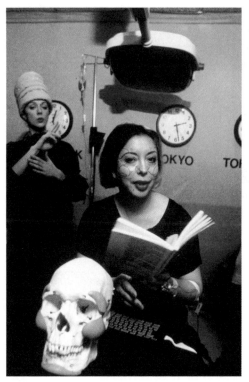

Figure 4 + 5. ORLAN, Seventh Surgery-Performance called *Omnipresence*, November 21, 1993, New York: *Skull with Blue implants, memento mori* and *Smile of Delight.* Cibachromes in diasec mount, 165x110 cm, Edition of 7 + 1. Photo Vladimir Sichov. © the artist and LACMA collection, Los Angeles, respectively/ billedkunst.dk.

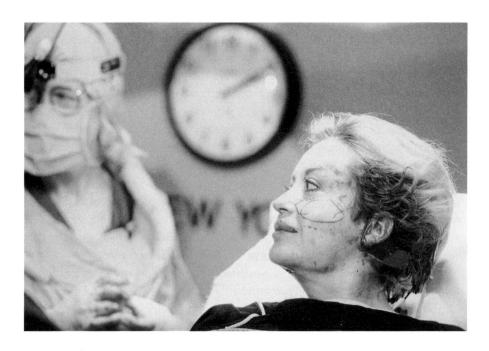

fulfilled in liberal democracy. As in some historical black hole, this Hegelian end of history – be it artistic or political – signifies an evolutionary fulfilment beyond which there is no future horizon to escape to. But how then is Fukuyama's 2002 book with its quite forward-looking title *Our Posthuman Future* to be understood? In it Fukuyama does address the technological means designed to temporarily or permanently change the human body: genetic modification, prosthetic enhancement, and intensification of perception, muscular strength and concentration through the use of drugs. While in a way seeing these technologies as having come to stay, and thus as something indeed qualifying a posthuman future for an "us" in the plural, Fukuyama nevertheless in practice advocates a hesitating procedure, based on the criteria of not a posthuman, but rather an emphatically human subject – one, however, whose fundamental characteristics, its human nature, are now just as much derived from Darwinian natural evolution as from its Hegelian cultural counterpart (2002: 130). Apart from pointing to infinite and to a large extent poorly understood and appreciated qualities of this human subject, Fukuyama foregrounds again that a basic quality of life, as we have come to know it, consists of dignity: a basic level of respect from our fellow beings (2002: 149). This dignity, also called Factor X, is actively sought for through recognition, sustained by, among other things, meritocracy. Can it, for instance, be truly satisfying to work if work is caused primarily by some technological enhancement of your body and not by your genetically determined talents or qualities meticulously obtained through education? Can it, specifically, be satisfying to make or contemplate a work of art, if the artist has not gone to a minimum amount of trouble to make it (2002: 149; oral statement by Fukuyama to author in the autumn of 2009)? Thus, in parallel to Danto's philosophical cloud, which protects the art object from becoming a mere thing – its thingness including non-trouble on the part of its 'maker' – Fukuyama wants to establish a state-sustained ethical apparatus to protect the human subject from becoming a mere automaton, an undignified being artificially upheld by posthuman enhancement.

Introducing the posthuman in evolution

The easiest way out of this historiographic impasse, blocking the future for both the political and aesthetic human being, is simply to abandon models pertaining to the philosophy of history and turn instead to utterly pragmatist statements like: the identity of the human has never been stable and we have, in a way, always been posthuman (Hayles 1999: 279; Halberstam and Livingston 1995: 8); or art makers do not care about the masochistic problems of art theoreticians (Belting 1987). My strategy here will, however, be the opposite; not weakening but expanding the philosophy of history. The problem seems to be how to save Hegel and yet move beyond him. In my own research into the evolution of pictorial space and landscape imagery, I can basically confirm the Hegelian model of aesthetical history prior to the twentieth century, according to which the evolution of self-consciousness, spirit, is mirrored in the arts moving from material to more ethereal media. Thus, in the pictorial arts up until 1900 the evolution of self-consciousness can be detected in an increasing marking out of a view point, an "I", positioning itself against an increasing depth-of-field (Wamberg 2009 [2005]). This directionality of human consciousness, moving towards ever-more autonomous stages of self-reflection, can even be conceived of as simply a continuation with new means of a tendency long under way in biological evolution, namely the interiorization of a steadily more autonomous virtual world in the animal brain and its sense apparatus (Huxley 1945 [1942]: 564-65) – what the Danish biosemiotician Jesper Hoffmeyer has termed "semiotic freedom" (Hoffmeyer and Favareau 2008 [2005]). Thus, whereas in nature this inner virtual world is evolved through anatomical changes in brains, in its cultural follower it is evolved in a macroscopically fixed brain, through microscopic specialization of brain centres resulting from specifically cultural means such as social exchange, practical experience and education.

The problem with the Hegelian explanation of consciousness is, however, that it posits the evolving human consciousness as its own driving force, indeed, as the name "world spirit" suggests, it amounts to a driving force of the world and of nature, which only becomes real through being perceived by consciousness. But how is this to make sense in a post-Darwinian world in which human self-consciousness is at best a late outcome of a natural evolution, which has generated its organisms through nearly four billion years without the intervention of anything that could be called consciousness? Neo-Darwinists such as Stephen Jay Gould (Gould, McGarr, and Rose 2007) and Daniel Dennett (1995: 320) solve the problem by simply denying the existence of such a thing as directionality in biological evolution, a process allegedly governed exclusively by accidental genetic mutations followed by natural selection. Hard pressed, Neo-Darwinists may state at most that rising complexity is purely an accidental outcome of this contingent interaction. However, if indeed we accept the evidence of directionality in both biological evolution and its cultural superstructure, it seems reasonable to suppose that it cannot be an accidental outcome of the blind watchmaker of natural selection; rather, it must be the result of an organizational force *upon which* natural selection operates, and which furthermore lies before and under the building up of that interiorized virtuality, which is eventually turning into self-consciousness. Literally, this directional tendency must be seen as a subconscious, self-organizational drive.

Theoretical framings that could expose such an evolutionary drive can be found in the recent meeting between biology and the trans-disciplinary sciences of complexity. According to theoreticians such as Kauffman (1995: 8), McShea and Bran-

148

don (2010) and Conway Morris (2003: 21), there is an emergent tendency towards rising complexity, an anti-entropic drive, in the open system of biological evolution. According to at least Kauffman, and to a lesser degree McShea and Brandon and Conway Morris, natural selection here functions not as the cause, but rather as an accompanying check of robustness, a devil's advocate in which the anti-entropic proposals are polished by entropy.

However, if we want to explore the role of culture in biology, and more specifically the pathway through which culture is now turning its own biological underpinnings into aggregates of nature and artifice, posthuman cyborgs, we should consult and elaborate on the continental philosophical tradition in which human consciousness and its cultural expressions do not only hover above and outside nature, as in Hegel, but rather emerge as phenomena fulfilling a drive that gradually comes into being in nature. Useful formulations for such a drive could be the spirit of nature moving from unconscious to conscious in the Romantic Schelling (Schelling 1978 [1800]); the will lying beneath and before its own distillate, the cognitive and virtual idea, in the Kantian follower Schopenhauer (1969 [1818]); or the *élan vital*, the organizational force leading into the organisms of biological evolution, in the French anti-dualist philosopher Bergson (1911 [1907]). The specifically posthuman lesson to extract from these philosophies would be one that Fukuyama in fact hints at at the end of his book (2002: 218):

> It may be that we are somehow destined to take up this new kind of freedom, or that the next stage of evolution is one in which, as some have suggested, we will deliberately take charge of our own biological makeup rather than leaving it to the blind forces of natural selection.

Accordingly, if the fundamental drive of organic nature is in fact not "the blind forces of natural selection" but an underlying force upon which natural selection operates and whose fundamental tendency is to transform itself into ever more complex stages of being, then human consciousness and its cultural products could be teleologically developed to function as a new and more efficient means of effecting that drive. This scenario, to be sure, in many ways resembles the progressive evolutionism of Pierre Teilhard de Chardin, the Jesuit palaeontologist who challenged Catholic orthodoxy by naturalizing Christian eschatological expectations. In Teilhard's spiritualist vision, though, technology paves the way for a collective consciousness, the so-called noosphere, which is still, Hegel fashion, somewhat separated from the materiality embedding it (Teilhard de Chardin 1969). In a truly posthuman perspective, however, consciousness and its products interfere so densely with nature that they can no longer be construed as standing outside their object but merge with its drive, which they are in fact fulfilling, in a hybrid venture, a posthuman co-genesis. In this perspective, the epoch of human consciousness and its cultural products emerge not so much as a separate history, which must be finished in an absolute endism, as is still the case in the Hegelianisms of Danto and Fukuyama; rather the human epoch shrinks to a parenthesis in natural history, a passage through which the subconscious drive of nature channels itself to a new and more complex stage, the posthuman. The posthuman, then, amounts to a post-conscious interlacing of consciousness and its cultural products into nature's subconscious.

Such a post-Hegelian philosophy of history would, of course, imply the risk of plunging into a too friction-less implementation of biotechnology: if it is a deep-lying desire of natural evolution to absorb technology as its new instrument of change, with the transformation of the human body into posthuman cyborg as a prime agenda, then what are we waiting for? Such a posthuman eagerness of human transformation, legitimizing itself based on a natural teleology, could easily re-awaken bad memories of Nazi eugenics, and to cool it a humanist scepticism like Fukuyama's, even when based on "obsolete" principles, would seem to be more efficient than a modified posthumanism. Nevertheless, even without the specifically posthuman discourse, it is my impression that humanism is today, ironically, in the process of being undermined by the ideology that otherwise sustains it in Fukuyama's Neo-Hegelian narrative: liberalist democracy. Absorbing a materialist utilitarianism, liberalist democracy is in danger of reducing the human subject to a labouring and consuming robot whose only raison d'être is on the one hand to participate in a work survival competition resembling the Darwinian struggle of existence, and on the other hand to have narcotic kicks in the likewise competitive "experience economy". Although termed "human", such a subject seems to be an even easier object for being upgraded according to materialist ideas of efficiency than a subject explicitly framed within a posthuman discourse.

The avant-gardes and nature's subconscious

It is against such a materialist version of posthumanism, forcing the subconscious drive of nature into a one-dimensional version of progress – plutocratic social Darwinism – that I think the experiences exposed in avant-garde art and aesthetics might be important, indeed highly needed. In Schelling, Schopenhauer and Bergson, art enjoys in fact a privileged position among the human areas of knowledge, precisely because it is in touch with the deeper-lying drives of nature, which are exposed through the artist's genius or intuition. Whereas the exact sciences and their accompanying logical philosophies analyse nature according to abstractions that are far removed from the world that they conceptualize, the arts unfold in a material embedding, which makes them more receptive to the creative forces of nature – forces that are likewise unfolding in matter. In Bergson's words (1911 [1907]: 177):

Our eye perceives the features of the living being, merely as assembled, not as mutually organized. ... This intention is just what the artist tries to regain, in placing himself back within the object by a kind of sympathy, in breaking down, by an effort of intuition, the barrier that space puts up between him and his model. It is true that this aesthetic intuition, like external perception, only attains the individual. But we can conceive an inquiry turned in the same direction as art, which would take life *in general* for its object, just as physical science, in following to the end the direction pointed out by external perception, prolongs the individual facts into general laws. (Bergson's italics)

However, a specifically posthuman elaboration of this sort of philosophy, which considers the arts as especially receptive to natural drives and therefore as prototypical of a more general inquiry into life's creativity, would nevertheless state that in the nineteenth century the arts also had become too removed from actual physical processes, which they contemplated only in the form of distant representations, as another version of physics' "external perception". According to such posthuman criticism, the whole avant-garde and modernist project could exactly be about returning the artistic and aesthetic experience of nature's subconscious to the actual world, transforming the arts into a huge laboratory of experiments for upcoming posthuman forms of life. Such an exposure of nature's subconscious in the physical surroundings would, for instance, be almost identical with the self-understanding of the Surrealists who conceived of Surrealism as a new realism in which the border between the subconscious and world, dream and reality, was erased (Breton 1985).

This avant-garde exposure of nature's subconscious should in no way imply a naïve return to nature. In fact, one of the shocks of avant-garde art has been its continual absorption of technology, mechanical repetition, scientific mapping, game rules and so forth; and an equally hesitant, almost paranoic attitude towards using organic elements or modelling the artwork according to organic principles. As was clearly sensed in Ortega (1948), and as repeated by theoreticians like Clement Greenberg (1986 [1939]) and Adorno (2002 [1970]: 66), organic elements, graphically displayed, turn art into kitsch. If this anti-organic and technological engagement is emblematic of the degree to which consciousness interlaces itself with the subconscious drives of nature in the posthuman context, nevertheless it also twists the rational contexts of technology's usual utilitarian contexts, opening up towards a more unpredictive and playful space, including coincidences, interactivity and other more open creative principles. According to the Situationists, for instance, art (the completely useless) and technology (the completely useful) should be re-integrated in a playful activity displacing the notion of work (Home 1996).

Confronted with this avant-garde engagement in technology and the physical world more generally, we could ask if artworks are at all in need of Danto's art philosophical cloud to protect them against becoming mere things? Are we not closer to Peter Bürger's reading, in which the cloud's base in the art institution emerges rather as a prison, preventing the avant-gardistic forces from spreading to and revolutionizing the world according to aesthetic principles? The solution is dependent on how much transformative power is ascribed to the artistic object itself: is it a weak prosaic object in need of philosophical nursing in a never-ending eve of art, or is it in itself laden with revolutionary energy that deserves to be released in a posthuman world – a world that perhaps no longer needs the art category at all, bound as it is to the human subject whose aesthetic reflection it is?

In our posthuman perspective the answer would probably be both/and. Although avant-garde art does introduce a more matter-bound dimension, this dimension is not to be separated from the reflective side, with which it establishes a new insoluble compound, a performative aggregate, which could exactly be termed posthuman. In high-modern philosophical theories like Descartes' and Kant's, consciousness and its outer representations in signs and their material base, the media, should be sharply separated from the physical world, *das Ding an sich*, to which they refer (Peirce 1931: 5-6). However, if the emergence of the posthuman truly signifies a post-conscious stage of evolution, a stage in which the border between spirit and matter is challenged, then we must assume that this nominalist gap between sign and thing is challenged in favour of a compound of sign and thing. This linking seems, indeed, to manifest itself with increasing force in the media, or rather post-media, technologies developed since the 19th century: photography and film with their indexical imprints of past objects, television with its indexical imprints from present objects, and the computer which may manipulate present objects through signs. These post-mediatic compounds make one understand the media theorist Marshall McLuhan's characterization of the electrical age as an exteriorization of the human nerve system (McLuhan 1964), because at least in prosthetic form they break down the barrier between inner virtual and outer real worlds. They also make one comprehend his notion of the electrical age as neo-primitive and mythical, since the computer's manipulation of material things through signs indeed resembles a restaging of magic, a performative practice, which one could define as exactly erasing the border between wishful concept and physical realization. My claim would then be that avant-garde art like Warhol's Brillo Boxes is deeply concerned with exploring this emerging posthuman performative dimension of signs, the flowing together of medium and thing, communicating and doing.

A later artistic example, which explores this post-media dimension explicitly in relation to new technologies and evolution – and which accordingly seems to be more obviously posthuman – is the Brazilian-American Eduardo Kac's installation *Genesis* (1999) (Kac 2005). Through several steps of translation, from English to morse to DNA, coli bacteria have had a genetic message inserted from Genesis, the passage in which God transfers his power over the animals and plants to man. Through sign manipulation on the internet, these bacteria can now be made accessible to remote viewers, who while seeing them through ultraviolet light, simultaneously trigger genetic reactions that corrupt the original genetic message of man's sovereignty over the natural world. Thus, not only are the boundaries between signalling and doing broken down, the question "who creates whom?" is made perfectly unanswerable. And so this work could be taken as an allegory of that co-evolutionary genesis, the posthuman, which is emerging from the formerly separated agents: human culture and biological evolution.

■ References

Adorno, Theodor W. 2002 [1970]. *Aesthetic theory*, eds. Gretel Adorno and Rolf Tiedemann. London: Continuum.

Belting, Hans. 1987. *The end of the history of art?* Chicago: The University of Chicago Press.

Bergson, Henri. 1911 [1907]. *Creative evolution*. Mineola, NY: Dover.

Breton, André. 1985. *Manifestes du surréalisme*. Paris: Gallimard.

Bürger, Peter. 1984 [1980, 1974]. *Theory of the avant-garde*. Minneapolis: University of Minnesota Press.

Conway Morris, Simon. 2003. *Life's solution: Inevitable humans in a lonely universe*. New York: Cambridge University Press.

Danto, Arthur C. 1997. *After the end of art: Contemporary art and the pale of history*. Princeton, NJ: Princeton University Press.

Danto, Arthur C. 1986. *The philosophical disenfranchisement of art*. New York: Columbia University Press.

Dennett, Daniel Clement. 1995. *Darwin's dangerous idea: Evolution and the meanings of life*. London: Penguin.

Fukuyama, Francis. 2002. *Our posthuman future: Consequences of the biotechnology revolution*. London: Profile.

Fukuyama, Francis. 1992. *The end of history and the last man*. New York: Avon Books.

Gould, Stephen Jay, Paul McGarr and Steven Rose. 2007. *The richness of life: The essential Stephen Jay Gould*. London: Vintage.

Greenberg, Clement. 1986 [1939]. "Avant-Garde and Kitsch", in *The collected essays and criticism*, ed. John O'Brian. Chicago: University of Chicago Press. Vol.1. 5-22.

Halberstam, Judith, and Ira Livingston (eds.). 1995. *Posthuman bodies*. Bloomington: Indiana University Press.

Hayles, N. Katherine. 1999. *How we became posthuman: Virtual bodies in cybernetics, literature, and informatics*. Chicago: University of Chicago Press.

Hegel, Georg Wilhelm Friedrich. 1975 [1835]. *Aesthetics: Lectures on fine art*. Trans. T.M. Knox. Oxford: Clarendon Press.

Hoffmeyer, Jesper and Donald Favareau. 2008 [2005]. *Biosemiotics: An examination into the signs of life and the life of signs*. Scranton, PA: University of Scranton Press.

Home, Stewart. 1996. *What is situationism? A reader*. Edinburgh: AK Press.

Huxley, Julian. 1945 [1942]. *Evolution, the modern synthesis*. London: Allen & Unwin.

Kac, Eduardo. 2005. *Telepresence and bio art: Networking humans, rabbits, and robots*. Ann Arbor: University of Michigan Press.

Kauffman, Stuart. 1995. *At home in the universe: The search for laws of self-organization and complexity.* London: Viking.

Kojève, Alexandre. 1969 [1947]. *Introduction to the reading of Hegel: Lectures on the Phenomenology of spirit.* New York: Basic Books.

McLuhan, Marshall. 1964. *Understanding media: The extensions of man.* New York: McGraw-Hill.

McShea, Daniel W. and Robert N. Brandon. 2010. *Biology's first law: The tendency for diversity and complexity to increase in evolutionary systems.* Chicago: University of Chicago Press.

Ortega y Gasset, José. 1948. *The dehumanization of art, and notes on the novel.* Trans. Helene Weyl. Princeton NJ: Princeton University Press.

Peirce, Charles Sanders. 1931. *Principles of philosophy. Collected papers of Charles Sanders Peirce*, Vol. 1, eds. Charles Hartshorne, Paul Weiss. Cambridge, MA: Harvard University Press.

Schelling, F.W.J. 1978 [1800]. *System of transcendental idealism.* Charlottesville, VA: University of Virginia Press.

Schopenhauer, Arthur. 1969 [1818]. *The world as will and representation.* New York: Dover.

Teilhard de Chardin, Pierre. 1969. *The future of man.* London: Fontana.

Wamberg, Jacob. 2009 [2005]. *Landscape as world picture: Tracing cultural evolution in images.* Aarhus: Aarhus University Press.

PART IV

POLITICAL POSSIBILITIES

11 Agency or Inevitability: Will Human Beings Control Their Technological Future?

Francis Fukuyama

Constant technological change has been a feature of human societies since the beginning of the Industrial Revolution, and technological revolutions have always brought with them enormous social consequences. The harnessing of steam power to iron and steel triggered industrialization itself; the scale economies of assembly-line manufacturing and the need for command-and-control networks created the modern city, promoting political centralization and planning (Beniger 1986); and the information and communications technology revolutions have tended to decentralize and make less expensive access to information, thereby aiding democracy.

The ongoing biotechnology revolution is already having enormous consequences for society. Whether this will be better or worse for human freedom and opportunity will depend not just on the technologies themselves, but on the governance mechanisms that human beings create to manage them. While science and technology will always advance in aggregate, human societies have demonstrated an ability to influence the rate of advance of particular technologies that are socially problematic, from nuclear weapons to toxic chemicals to disease agents. But the degree of control that can be exercised depends on the nature of the technology, the uses people make of it, and the interaction effects concerned (President's Council 2004).

Future biotechnologies promise great benefits to human health and happiness, and there is thus a general presupposition that advances in this field are a good thing socially. Before we can talk about regulating biotechnology, however, we need to discuss what sorts of human goods are at stake that might require such intervention (Fukuyama and Furger 2006).

What's Wrong with Human Redesign?

Human biomedicine was seen from the beginning as having potentially problematic effects, which is why there are bioethics councils everywhere but no info-ethics equivalents. Human biotechnology raises different issues from those brought on by agricultural biotech. Some people argue that the main danger posed by biotech is its use by potentially tyrannical governments, but that if choices are freely made by informed adults or acting on their own or on behalf of their children, there is no problem. Even under these circumstances, however, there are potential harms that can be placed into three categories: (1) utilitarian concerns, (2) ambiguity as to what constitutes human "improvement", based on a failure to understand human complexity; and finally (3) moral issues regarding manipulation of what constitutes a human essence. We will deal with each of these in turn.

■ Utilitarian issues

There are a number of purely utilitarian issues raised by innovation and experimentation in biotechnology. The simplest and most straightforward has to do with safety. The history of pharmaceutical innovation is littered with cases of unintended side effects, many of which have appeared only years after a drug was introduced. Given the complexity of human genetic causation – that is, the interactions between genes and environment, and genes with each other – it is very difficult to predict the effects of a given genetic manipulation. Germ-line modification and reproductive cloning are by definition experiments that would be carried out on subjects who cannot give informed consent (i.e., the unborn), and therefore would violate prima facie the rules set down in the Helsinki Declaration for human subject research (McNeill 1993: 54-55). While we could assume that parents might be willing to take risks on behalf of their children, it would be much easier to accept these risks were the intervention's purpose a therapeutic one, for example to correct a severe genetic disorder like Tay-Sachs. Germ-line experimentation for enhancement purposes would be far more problematic.

A second issue has to do with negative externalities, which is a standard social situation calling for state regulation. There are many biomedical interventions that would make sense from an individual standpoint, but which are in aggregate socially harmful.

We already have an ongoing example of this, which is sex selection, a practice that has taken place in certain Asian countries when parents were given access to technologies that could determine the sex of a fetus *in utero* (Schenker 2002; Ansari-Lari and Saadat 2002; Chan et al. 2002; Stephen 2000). In countries which have a cultural preference for boys, the selective abortion of female fetuses may make sense for individual families, but for society as a whole it leads to skewed sex ratios and down the road a surplus of males in a given age cohort. There are many reasons for thinking that a population of unmarriageable males would produce negative social effects like increased crime and political instability. Hence what makes sense for individual parents doesn't necessarily make sense for society as a whole.

Another technological possibility that would be individually but not socially desirable is life extension (Fukuyama 2002: 57-71). Many people dream of a breakthrough that would allow them to live to the age of 150 or 200 years, but from the standpoint of society as a whole there are a number of reasons for thinking that this would not be a good idea. These reasons have to do with the functions of death and generational turnover as general adaptive mechanisms, and why evolution hasn't given humans the lifespan of bristlecone pines already. Human beings need relatively long life spans compared to most mammals to raise and train their young, given their cognitive abilities and body mass. But skills eventually deteriorate, habits become ingrained, and it is generally easier to raise and train a new human being rather than having an older one adapt. For populations, generational replacement is clearly a good thing; it keeps both skills and social arrangements fresh, and permits institutional adaptation.

Moreover, when people envision life extension for themselves, they have in mind a younger version of themselves that is being kept alive, and don't think seriously about the tradeoff between quantity and quality of life that is inevitably involved. The life extension revolution is already playing out in nursing homes around the world. By the time human beings reach their mid-80s, roughly half are subject to degenerative diseases like Parkinson's and Alzheimer's; what contemporary biomedicine has allowed them to do is to die slowly over a period of years rather than dying quickly from a heart attack or cancer. Of course, future breakthroughs in medicine will potentially allow us to prevent or cure such degenerative diseases. But in order for life extension to avoid a scenario in which a substantial portion of the elderly population is living in a prolonged state of dependence, one would have to imagine a world in which people's different life systems would shut down quickly and in close unison, rather then being sequenced over a number of years. My personal bet is that this isn't likely to happen.

Changes in birthrates coupled with extended life spans brought about by already existing biomedical technologies have already created a crisis of sustainability in many advanced societies. Total fertility rates in Japan, Korea, Taiwan, China, Singapore, Italy, Spain, and other places have fallen dramatically, and in some countries these rates are just half of replacement rates. These societies are undergoing a process of depopulation unprecedented in human history, apart from disasters brought on by disease, famine, and war. It has been reliably predicted that the population of Japan will fall by about one-third by the middle of the 21st century. The dependency ratio is shifting from four workers for every retired person ten years ago to two by this same period (Eberstadt 1997: 3-22). Future advances in biomedicine have and will ease this problem by allowing older people to keep working for much longer than in the past, but an equally likely outcome is to actually increase dependency ratios by making possible more expensive end-of-life interventions.

The impending future, in which population distributions look not like pyramids but like trapezoids resting on small bases, can theoretically be managed through changes in various social institutions. Existing social contracts that underpin modern welfare states were written back in an age in which life expectancies were 20 years lower and birth rates twice as high; consumption will have to fall and savings rates will have to rise dramatically. There is already huge political resistance to making these shifts, however: Nicolas Sarkozy's government faced weeks of strikes and social protest at the idea of raising the retirement age from 60 to 62. It is not sufficient to say that taxes will have to rise to cover these costs; tax rates in a country like Japan would have to be so high that they would undermine prospects for economic growth. Another way of easing the problem would be to permit greater immigration from parts of the world that haven't undergone the demographic transition yet; but immigration also produces political backlash and cultural conflict. Longer working lives would have to be accommodated by periodic retraining and downward social mobility on the part of aging workers; this too is possible but implies a very different world than the one mankind has been living in up to now. Medical treatments for people nearing the end of life would have to be strictly rationed in order to avoid robbing the young of their futures to pay for the old. Politically, however, any talk of rationing is at present totally unacceptable; look at the hysteria caused during the US healthcare reform debate over the charge that the Obama administration was planning to institute "death panels".

The reason I am discussing the social impact of life extension is that these scenarios do not depend on dramatic breakthroughs in synthetic biology or some other science fiction scenario. They are already playing out: Japan is the country furthest along in this social crisis and will act as the canary in the coal mine for other societies. Demography, unlike other social science disciplines, can make fairly reliable predictions about the future, and this is one that is upon us already given past advances in biomedicine. Should the aggregate impact of new technological innovations in synthetic biology extend human life expectancies by another decade – something which seems entirely within the realm of possibility – the social crisis will be even worse.

■ The failure to understand complexity

A second reason for being cautious about the use of biomedical technologies to modify human behavior has to do with a lack of understanding of what constitutes human improvement, which is ultimately related to the failure to understand complexity in human evolution. Many people believe that the targets of such interventions would be unambiguous goods, like greater intelligence, freedom from genetic diseases, lesser predisposition towards violence and criminality, longevity, and the like. The problem is one of unanticipated consequences when seeking to change enormously complex systems. We have already seen how increased longevity is desirable on an individual level, but possibly harmful on a social level. There are some other examples as well.

There is evidence that homosexuality is a genetically-caused phenomenon, and that it is affected by the levels of testosterone to which fetuses are exposed *in utero*. It is perfectly possible to imagine medical interventions in which pregnant women could not only predict the likelihood that their unborn children were gay, but also affect the outcome itself. Were it to be possible for parents to affect the sexual orientation of their children, would that constitute human "improvement"? Were such a procedure to become widely used and lead to a sharp reduction in the proportion of gays and lesbians within a given society, would that society be better off? How would this change affect the interests and moral standing of those who remained? Similarly, if parents could choose the skin pigmentation or racial/ethnic features of their unborn children, would we regard this as an uncontroversial expansion of individual choice, or as a potentially divisive trend socially (Elliot 2003: 191-193)?

Other types of interventions targeting behavioral traits like aggression, propensity towards violence, alcoholism, and the like are similarly problematic. These propensities have evolved in human beings over a period of millions of years in order to permit the species to survive, and are linked to survival chances in ways that may not at first seem evident. In human evolution, for example, competitiveness and aggression are intimately linked to the development of cooperative skills; human beings cooperate in order to compete, and compete in order to cooperate. If parents or a society decide for moral or ideological reasons that they want kinder or gentler children or, conversely, tougher and more aggressive ones (whether through the use of drugs, or through a germ-line intervention), they may be surprised to find their children disadvantaged in unexpected ways. A society that in the aggregate opts for one or another choice may find itself in an unexpectedly difficult position when dealing with other societies that have made different choices.

■ Human nature and human rights

A final reason to be cautious about the use of new biomedical technologies to alter human behavior, particularly through germ-line engineering, has to do with the nature of political rights. Modern understandings of human rights are based on a certain essentialist view of human nature. Even though Darwinism postulates that such an essence does not exist, our moral system in fact depends on a belief in the existence of a universal human essence that gives us, as opposed to non-human animals or inanimate natural objects, political rights. Some reference to human rights and human dignity is written into the constitutions or fundamental laws of most modern liberal democracies. We are allowed to use animals for food, and to experiment upon them without their consent, because we believe that they have a lesser dignity than do human beings. We do not discriminate based on race, ethnicity, or gender because we believe that people who differ according to these biological characteristics nonetheless possess a common human essence. We argue that skin color is not an essential characteristic of human beings. Though we are loath to define too categorically what does constitute that essence, there is a rich discussion in different religious and philosophical traditions as to what it is. In the Western tradition, it has something to do with the human ability to act as moral agents, to reason and use language, and to empathize. We deny full political rights to those in the human community who do not share these characteristics fully, like children, the criminally insane, or elderly people who have lost certain vital faculties (Fukuyama 2001; Schulz and Fukuyama 2002: 113-123).

It stands to reason, then, that if we develop a biotechnology that is powerful enough to affect that essence, we will also be affecting the nature of rights. What happens when we are able to insert non-human genes into human beings to give them new characteristics that no human being has had before? Or what would happen if an animal is given human genes, to give it faculties that someone regards as desirable? What would the political rights of such hybrid creatures be?

One great fear that many people rightly have about future potential uses of bio-technology is that it will be used by elites to genetically embed certain advantages like intelligence, good looks, or athletic ability. Those with resources and education are likely to be early adopters of new enhancement technologies, and given the competitiveness of today's elites, one suspects that parents may be forced into this kind of competition even if they have moral qualms about it. In some sense, these kinds of inequalities are already being bred into modern societies; with women receiving higher levels of education, assortative mating ensures that the children of elite couples are likely to be born with genetic advantages. In the days when Europe was a class-based society, people of lower social orders looked physically different from elites, because they had significantly poorer diets and healthcare. Higher living standards and better access to education revealed to people that class differences were socially constructed, which paved the way for the modern egalitarian understanding of rights. The deliberate introduction of genetic stratification of human societies will inevitably force societies to rethink this issue.

Governing Technology

Can and should science be regulated? There is a widespread view held by many intelligent people that this is (a) normatively wrong and (b) impossible to implement in practice. Many believe that modern natural science is a self-contained and self-justifying system that ought to be shielded from politics. As then-congressman Ted Strickland said in the US debate on a proposed cloning ban: "We should not allow theology, philosophy, or politics to interfere with the decision we make on this issue [of a cloning ban]". There is a strong techno-libertarian position that sees efforts to regulate new biotechnologies as a modern-day instance of the Catholic Church's efforts to stifle Galileo, something wrong and ultimately futile.

Societies regulate science and technology all the time, however, and do so quite legitimately. Let's begin with the normative issue. In the realm of science, who is sovereign and gets to decide what can and can't be done? The answer under virtually any version of modern democratic theory would be that the people constituting a society are sovereign and that they alone have the legitimate right to put limits on activities undertaken in their societies. Modern natural science does not carve out a separate normative domain where it sets its own standards for right and wrong. Congressman Strickland had it exactly wrong: it is not scientists, but rather theologians, philosophers, and politicians who have the ultimate authority to place limits on scientific research. Societies desiring the benefits of science may decide to delegate large amounts of discretion to epistemic communities to manage their own affairs, but this makes them morally and politically subsidiary to the larger community (Fukuyama and Furger 2006: 42).

If one doubts the truth of this, one has only to consider the matter of human experimentation. A number of the horrifying experiments carried out in the United States, such as Willowbrook (when children were deliberately injected with hepatitis), or the Tuskegee experiments (when poor black men were not treated for syphilis in a controlled trial), as well as experiments by Nazi scientists, actually constituted good science methodologically, whose results could potentially be used for good ends like fighting disease (McNeill 1993: 61-63). Contemporary rules requiring informed consent on the part of the subjects of human experimentation were imposed politically on the scientific community by the larger national and world communities, and are embodied in international standards like the Nuremburg Code and the Helsinki Declaration. Biomedicine would advance much more quickly if we could use human beings the way we use laboratory mice, but we choose a slower rate of advance because we want to protect certain basic human values. So the principle of political control is well established.

While many people seem to think that the regulation of biotechnology would be a novel thing, the fact is that human biomedicine is already one of the most heavily regulated areas of science and technology development (Fukuyama and Furger 2006). What is more novel is regulation not out of a concern for safety and efficacy, which guide institutions like the US Food and Drug Administration, but regulation on ethical grounds. Institutions like the US National Institutes of Health already allocate research funds based on ethical considerations having to do with embryo politics, a situation imposed on them by various Congressional mandates. But other countries have designed regulatory institutions with the sole purpose of looking closely at the ethical issues raised by novel biotechnologies. One of these is the British Human Fertilisation and Embryology Authority (HFEA), which created a review board structure that includes lay members to look at experimentation and clinical practice in reproductive medicine.[1] Other countries including Canada, Australia, and France have set up similar organizations (Fukuyama and Furger 2006: 149-181 and appendix H).

The design of such organizations needs to be carefully thought through. On first blush, it might seem appropriate to simply expand the authority of existing food and drug regulators to cover ethical issues as well, as the US FDA has already tried to do in the case of human reproductive cloning. There are a number of good reasons to prefer the creation of an entirely new organization with its own mandate, however. Existing bureaucracies have their own internal culture and history, and they often find it difficult to take on new tasks. The US Interstate Commerce Commission (ICC) was established in the 19th century to regulate railroads; when interstate trucking became a common practice this activity was added to its regulatory mandate. The economics of rail carriage and trucking are quite different, however, and the skills shaped in one context did not lend themselves to the other. The ICC could have become the regulator of airlines as well when they started to fly between states, but the earlier poor experiences with trucking regulation convinced people that this new form of transportation needed its own regulatory authority, the Federal Aviation Administration (FAA). So too in the case of biotechnology: a regulatory agency devoted to, say, reproductive medicine would need to focus on one clearly defined area of technology development, and have a mandate that would allow it to include ethical considerations in its decision-making, and not simply issues related to safety and efficacy. It is not clear that this is a function that can simply be added to the mandate of existing regulators.

---

1. The HFEA grew out of the Report of the Committee of Inquiry into Human Fertilisation and Embryology, Cm 9314, July 1984, also known as the Warnock report.

■ The general problem of regulation

Whatever a society decides to regulate, it gets less of. Since everyone would agree that we want to have vigorous innovation in human biomedicine, we would want a regulatory system that both encourages innovation and the development of new medicines and techniques, but that also observes socially-determined ethical boundaries both in research methods and in outcomes.

Regulatory agencies receive a mandate that grants them a degree of discretion, hopefully well-defined in the enabling legislation, to make detailed decisions in implementing the legislature's will. Governments can also regulate science and technology through their funding decisions; in the United States, an agency like the National Institutes of Health has enormous influence over what is and is not studied in the life sciences. In virtually all cases, regulatory or funding authority requires the delegation of decision-making powers to the epistemic community that is responsible for technological advance in the particular area being regulated. In an extremely fast-moving area of science, that delegation has to be very substantial.

The trick in designing a good regulatory system is to avoid both the excessive politicization of decisions, as well as blanket grants of authority to the epistemic communities in question. One does not want Congress to determine exactly how many parts per million of a particular toxin constitutes an unsafe level; on the other hand, one would not consider delegating the decision of how to treat human embryos to a technical agency. Large and controversial decisions like the moral status of embryos are obviously political ones that have to be played out in political arenas like Congress.

In addition, one would like a regulatory body to be deliberative and not simply subject to interest group pressure. In the United States, administrative agencies are subject to the 1946 Administrative Practices Act, which supposedly seeks public input through postings of new regulations in the Federal Register and the solicitation of public notice-and-comment. In practice, however, this process has been dominated by well-organized interest groups that may represent small parts of the public, which nonetheless are capable of shaping or blocking legislation in ways that would not necessarily be supported by public opinion. This is one of the reasons why the United States has not been able to pass a reproductive cloning ban since such legislation was first attempted in the early 2000s: both the pro-life and scientific/industry communities were sufficiently well-organized to prevent the passage of compromise legislation that would for example have prohibited reproductive cloning while permitting certain forms of research cloning (Fukuyama and Furger 2006: 245-291).

If new regulatory bodies were to be created to deal with some of the ethical concerns noted above, how would they seek to limit new technologies? Obviously, this is something that could only be decided through a democratic process in which legislatures and publics informed themselves sufficiently about the underlying issues and laid down broad guidelines for regulatory agencies. Obviously those guidelines would differ from one society to another. German and Canadian regulators do not permit embryonic stem cell research, while British ones do. Whatever one's moral givens, the actual rules laid down would necessarily have to reflect a democratic consensus.

One general way to frame future regulation that would encompass many of the utilitarian and moral concerns raised above would be to have the regulatory authority distinguish between therapeutic and enhancement technologies, and to either ban the latter, make them substantially more expensive, or otherwise restrict access to them. It would seem quite reasonable to say that in a world where millions of people do not have basic healthcare, investment resources ought to go to innovative treatments for the sick, rather than enhancements that will allow the already rich and healthy to make their lives even better. While many people would argue that it is not theoretically possible to draw a clear distinction between therapy and enhancement, such distinctions are made all the time in the world of drug regulation, and are eminently something that a regulatory agency could be tasked to do (President's Council 2003).

International Considerations

Many people argue that it is pointless to try to regulate human biomedicine on a national basis, since globalization and international competition mean that another country will simply seek to undertake the banned or regulated activity. This argument has been made repeatedly during the US stem cell debate, and indeed certain Asian countries like China and Singapore have seen American moral compunctions on embryo research as giving them a competitive opening. In general there is no question that technologies, expertise, and people cross borders very easily now, especially in an area like biotechnology that does not depend on large-scale economies or heavy government subsidies.

There are indeed a number of cultural differences between societies that lead to very different stances on biomedical research. Western views on human dignity find their origins in Judaeo-Christian doctrine, which accords human beings a special and higher dignity than the rest of natural creation, and awards man the right to dominion over nature. Asian moral doctrines like Buddhism, Shinto, or Daoism, by contrast, do not make such strong dichotomous distinctions between human and non-human nature, seeing nature rather as a continuum in which spiritual life can exist in non-human beings. This perspective has led to perhaps a gentler and less exploitative attitude towards the natural world, but also to an arguably less protective attitude towards human life as such. This is reflected above all in lower levels of moral opposition in Asian societies to abortion and infanticide. Except in countries like Korea where Christianity has made inroads, embryonic stem cell research has simply not been as controversial there as in America or parts of Europe.

The degree to which the present globally distributed system of science and technology development undermines the possibilities for regulation depends on exactly what is being regulated. In areas where safety and efficacy are concerned, like drug development, internationalization has not led to a regulatory "race to the bottom"; indeed, strict regulatory environments like that of the United States often give pharmaceutical companies that develop products under them competitive advantages. Relaxed regulatory standards become a competitive advantage only when cost becomes a critical factor, such as the manufacturing of generic drugs for sale in very poor countries.

One challenging area for international regulation concerns synthetic biology, and its potential use to create new biological weapons that could be used either by states or by terrorist organizations. Unlike nuclear weapons, which are very capital-intensive to produce, bioengineering can increasingly be done on a small scale with readily available equipment. Like nuclear weapons, it is possible to conceive of a single laboratory escaping regulatory control and producing a dangerous virus or microbe that could do substantial damage to large numbers of people, increasing the need for a leak-proof system (Specter 2009).

In other areas like enhancement technologies targeting human capabilities or behavior, the regulatory challenge is in a sense much less severe. If the major objections to biomedical interventions were primarily ethical, the fact that such things were being done in other countries would not undermine the logic of continuing to regulate them in one's own society. In a way the situation would be comparable to safety and health regulation: other countries may have laxer standards with regard to these issues and derive some competitive advantage from that fact, but are not for that reason widely imitated by countries with higher standards. Only if a particular enhancement technology seems to provide a clear national advantage – for instance something that affects national security or economic competitiveness – would there be strong pressures to follow suit internationally.

An obvious answer to the problem posed by globalization would be to coordinate national regulation through some form of international agreement or organization. This has been tried already in a limited way, in the form of a United Nations-sponsored ban on reproductive cloning, which several European countries proposed in the early 2000s. It failed for the same reasons that similar legislation failed in the United States: pro-life groups that would have normally supported a reproductive cloning ban were opposed to a ban that did not simultaneously ban research cloning, for fear that their action would legitimate the latter. It is hard to see how international regulation will come about when the world's richest and most powerful country, the United States, has not been able to decide on a system of national regulation for itself. This is doubly so in an area where many countries are using their regulatory environment to create competitive niches for themselves.

Conclusions

At the moment of the introduction of any new technology, contemporary commentators conclude that its progress is proceeding so rapidly and its newness is so much outside existing paradigms that it will never be susceptible to regulation. As Deborah Spar and Tim Wu have shown, this was true not just of the Internet, but also of older technologies like the telephone, telegraph, radio, and satellite TV (Spar 2001; Wu 2010). The reason that this happens is that the initial pace of technological change far outstrips the rate of social adjustment. Over time, however, the rate of technological development slows, governance institutions catch up, and an uneasy balance is struck between innovation and social control. Despite early claims that the Internet could not be regulated, censors in China have been relatively successful in shutting down politically subversive web sites and preventing criticism of the regime from appearing there. In the years following Hiroshima and Nagasaki, specialists argued that several dozen countries would come to possess nuclear weapons in the coming decades, and that they would be routinely used in warfare. And yet, nearly 70 years after the end of World War II, nuclear weapons are owned by a small handful of countries, and none have been detonated in anger.

No system of social control is perfect. The barriers to nuclear proliferation erected in the 1960s and 70s are breaking down, and it may well be that the coming generation will see a nuclear weapon detonated in an act of war. But the fact that the rate of proliferation could be slowed for such a long time was an undoubted boon, and proves that some degree of governance of the direction of technological development is possible.

It is by no means inevitable that we will experience a "posthuman" future. The human goods at stake are sufficiently important that societies will proceed carefully in making use of new biotechnologies. It may be true that whatever can be done will eventually be done by someone, but it is important to our societies whether this happens tomorrow, or in a couple of generations. Rather than speaking abstractly about the possibilities of human agency, it is more urgent to think concretely about public policies that will allow us to enjoy the benefits of new technologies, and yet steer resources and talent into areas approved by a clear and stable social consensus.

References

Ansari-Lari, M. and M. Saadat. 2002. 'Changing Sex Ratios in Iran 1976-2000', in *Journal of Epidemiology and Community Health* 56.

Beniger, James R. 1986. *The Control Revolution: Technological and Economic Origins of the Information Society*. Cambridge: Harvard University Press.

Chan, Cecilia L.W. et al. 2002. 'Gender Selection in China: Its Meanings and Implications', in *Journal of Assisted Reproduction and Genetics* 19, no. 9.

Eberstadt, Nicholas. 1997. 'World Population Implosion?', in *Public Interest*, no. 129.

Elliott, Carl. 2003. *Better Than Well: American Medicine Meets the American Dream*. New York: W.W. Norton & Company.

Fukuyama, Francis and Franco Furger. 2006. *Beyond Bioethics: A Proposal for Modernizing the Regulation of Human Biotechnologies*. Washington D.C.: School of Advanced International Studies, Johns Hopkins University.

Fukuyama, Francis. 2001. 'Natural Rights and Human History", in *The National Interest*, no. 64.

Fukuyama, Francis. 2002. *Our Posthuman Future: Consequences of the Biotechnology Revolution*. New York: Farrar, Straus, and Giroux.

McNeill, Paul M. 1993. *The Ethics and Politics of Human Experimentation*. Cambridge: Cambridge University Press.

President's Council on Bioethics. 2003. *Beyond Therapy: Biotechnology and the Pursuit of Happiness*. Washington D.C.

President's Council on Bioethics. 2004. *Reproduction and Responsibility: The Regulation of New Biotechnologies*. Washington D.C.

Schenker, Joseph G. 2002. 'Gender Selection: Cultural and Religious Perspectives', in *Journal of Assisted Reproduction and Genetics* 19, no. 9.

Schulz, William and Francis Fukuyama. 2002. 'The Ground and Nature of Human Rights', in *The National Interest* no. 68.

Spar, Debora L. 2001. *Ruling the Waves: Cycles of Discovery, Chaos, and Wealth from the Compass to the Internet*. New York: Harcourt, Inc.

Specter, Michael. 2009. 'A Life of Its Own: Where Will Synthetic Biology Lead Us?' *The New Yorker*, Sept. 28.

Stephen, Elizabeth Hervey. 2000. 'Demographic Implications of Reproductive Technologies', in *Population Research and Policy Review*, no. 4.

Wu, Tim. 2010. *The Master Switch: The Rise and Fall of Information Empires*. New York: Knopf.

12 Biological Egalitarianism: A Defence

Torbjörn Tännsjö

Introduction[1]

Biological egalitarianism is the view that, biologically speaking, in all important respects human beings are equal. No matter how we conceive of the importance of various different biological aspects, this seems to me to be false, and I will explain in more detail below how I think it is false. However, conceived of rather as a normative than a descriptive view, biological egalitarianism has something going for it. At least it seems that we ought, if possible, to level out some biological differences in some important respects between people. In particular, this is something we should do with regard to our *cognitive* capacities, or so I will argue in this chapter.

The idea that we should level out differences between people with regard to cognitive capacities is not quite new. It has been hinted at by, for example, Francis Fukuyama, in his book, *Our Posthuman Future. Consequences of the Biotechnology Revolution*:

> Nobody knows whether genetic engineering will one day become as cheap and accessible as sonograms and abortion ... The most common fear expressed by present-day bioethicists is that only the wealthy will have access to this kind of genetic technology. But if a biotechnology of the future produces, for example, a safe and effective way to genetically engineer most intelligent children, then the stakes would immediately be raised. Under this scenario it is entirely plausible that an advanced, democratic welfare state would reenter the eugenics game, intervening this time not to prevent low-IO people from breeding, but to help genetically disadvantaged people to raise their IQs and the IQs of their offspring. (Fukuyama 2002: 81)

Even though this possibility is contemplated by Fukuyama, it is clear from the context that this is not something the author would favour. No rationale behind a rejection of the idea is provided in the book, however. As a matter of fact, many

---

1. A first draft of this paper was presented orally at the Aarhus conference "The Posthuman Condition" on 27 May 2010. A second version was presented to the seminar at Stockholm University on 26 October 2010, where Jonas Olson acted as my opponent. I thank him as well as the other participants in the seminar for many valuable comments.

of the arguments in the book could very well be used to *defend* such an application. I have myself suggested that it *might* be a good idea to level out our cognitive capacities (Tännsjö 2009: 421-432). What I will do here is to deal with this idea in greater detail.

My main objective in this chapter is to focus on this theme – not to examine in detail the argument of Fukuyama's book; however, I will point out the way in which I think the main thrust of the argument of Fukuyama's book really provides an independent argument in defence of the idea.

How could we establish biological cognitive equality? For the sake of simplicity, I will only discuss germ-line genetic engineering as the method to use in obtaining biological equality. I realise that in the future other means may exist as well, and indeed some of these exist already (pre-implantation genetic diagnostics, for instance). Furthermore, even more efficient drugs may be discovered which are capable of improving our capacity to stay focused, and perhaps even some drugs enhancing our capacity to remember. Germ-line genetic engineering will probably present us with the most radical possibilities if we want to improve our cognitive capacities in the future, however, and, anyway, what I say about germ-line genetic engineering is easily generalised to other methods. That's why I will say no more about them.

Before going into the argument for my thesis, I have to render it more precise, however.

Some Distinctions

It is helpful roughly (very roughly) to distinguish between three types of germ-line genetic engineering. First of all, we can use the method to exchange healthy alleles for sick ones, thereby preventing the occurrence of disease. This can be referred to as negative intervention or *gene therapy*. Secondly, we can use it in order to raise a person who is below a species mean to a high position, while staying within the special typical range. This can be referred to as positive intervention. Finally, we can use the method in order to improve some capacity *beyond* the species range, which can be referred to as enhancement (Tännsjö 1993: 231-247).

The third idea, what I call enhancement, is the main target of the argument in Fukuyama's book – hence its title. Here I will concede that, at least with respect to our cognitive capacities, there is no reason to try to enhance them. I have argued this point elsewhere, and I will not return to it here. So I leave cognitive enhancement to one side in the present context.

I will also set to one side the therapeutic (negative) use of germ-line genetic engineering. Even if it is anathema to all present international conventions on human rights and medicine and the like, this is something I am sure will take place in the future, and it is also something I believe most people will welcome, once it constitutes a safe possibility. So my exclusive interest here lies in positive interventions, i.e. the use of germ-line genetic engineering with regard to cognitive capacities to raise individuals from a low to a higher position – and yet leaving them within the *normal* human range. If we want to create more equal biological traits among people, it is the *positive* version of germ-line genetic engineering we should use.

The idea I will focus on, then, is the idea that we should level out our cognitive capacities by a policy of levelling up, but one where we stay within the species-typical variation. Since I am interested in equality (in the sense of narrowing the gap between those who perform best and those who are least intelligent), this means that we must set our target as high as possible within the species-normal variation. This does not only present an attractive ideal (as I will try to show), it also presents a clearly feasible one. It is hard to tell whether we will ever be capable of enhancing, in a safe manner, our cognitive capacities through germ-line genetic engineering, but it is not at all far-fetched to assume that we will be able to level out many differences among us. When we level up we work with genes, and combinations of genes, that exist in our common human gene pool and with which we are familiar; we do not construct new ones. This means less science fiction, of course, than if we were to construct *new* capacities that had never been heard of before.

Now, there is more than one way of establishing biological equality (to narrow the gap) with regard to cognitive capacities. One possibility is to attempt to give each person at least one important capacity at a high level. Then one would render true the false but common belief that those who are not talented at all in one field can always compensate for this by turning to another field, where they are truly talented. The common idea, then, is that each and any one of us can excel in at least one field. This is not true, since there seems to exist a positive correlation between the lack of various different talents; through germ-line genetic engineering, however, we could *render* it true.

However, I think the idea that each of us should be given at least one talent is extremely difficult to implement. Once the method is there, once a talent can be given to a prospective child, and once it is given to some prospective children, it becomes irresistible for you to give it to your own child as well, I submit. So I will only discuss the idea that we should level up in all possible cognitive dimensions.

Why level up, and not down, if we are interested in equality? Even if I think there is much to be said for a policy of levelling down, I will not discuss this possibility in the present chapter. I know that there are a lot of strong feelings ready to be called forth against the idea of levelling down, so even if such a policy were desirable it seems unlikely that it will ever happen; hence there is little interest in discussing it in the present context. I leave this discussion for another occasion.

I hold a rather broad and open view on what should count as a cognitive capacity. I am thinking here of our capacity to remember, both long term and short term, our capacity to stay focused when solving a problem, our intelligence as measured by an IQ test, our access to the world through our ordinary senses, our talent for drawing, our talent for music, including a good if not a perfect pitch, and so forth. I include also linguistic abilities and abilities to sympathise, and socialise, with others.

Human nature and moral theory

Human germ-line genetic engineering of the *enhancement* variety has sometimes been thought of as creating a threat to the moral standing of the creatures thus created. Or, more often, as creating a threat to those who have not been enhanced and who are therefore regarded as lagging behind. Is this problem genuine? It depends, of course, on what grants moral standing in the first place. Here it is convenient to consider three different approaches: (i) what I will call the 'humans are special' view, according to which mere membership of the human species grants human individuals the moral standing they have, (ii) what I will call, and what is often called, the moral rights idea that individuals have to qualify individually for moral standing by having certain cognitive capacities, and (iii) the utilitarian idea that individuals must be sentient (capable of feeling pleasure and pain) in order to possess moral standing. On all these three accounts, once you possess moral standing you must be taken into moral account. The *way* you are taken into account varies, of course, between these three moral traditions

Where does this place our suggestion that we should level out differences between people? Levelling out seems to be unproblematic from the point of view of the first idea of moral standing. When we level out we stay within the ordinary species typical range; hence, we do not create any individuals who are not truly human. Cognitive *enhancement* may mean that we create posthuman or transhuman individuals, who are not members of our species. Since what I here defend is a policy of levelling up, within our normal species boundaries, it will not create any individuals alien to us; so there is no need to go deeply into the question of whether this would be problematic or not, given the idea that human beings are special.

The moral rights idea that one must individually exhibit certain cognitive capacities in order to qualify for moral standing *is* of some relevance in the present context, however. At least it is relevant if the hurdle at which you gain moral standing (and moral rights) is fairly high. Then we may wonder whether all human beings qualify.

If some human beings don't qualify, this leads to an interesting question: should we do anything about it? Should we try to level up?

This idea that in order to have moral standing you must qualify individually is typical of moral rights theories. As I understand Fukuyama, he belongs to this tradition. There are two ways of conceiving of it. This theory could be taken to allow that there is a moral hierarchy where ordinary persons are morally superior to non-human animals, and superhuman individuals morally superior to us. Robert Nozick has toyed with this idea, but there is no necessity for a moral rights theorist to adopt it. A moral rights theorist may well argue more ecumenically that once you have leaped over the hurdle you possess full moral standing; all moral subjects are equal and no moral subjects are more equal than any others. Since I do not advocate the creation of superhuman creatures, I need not go any further into the distinction between the hierarchical and the ecumenical version of the moral rights theory. Note, however, that in both versions it is possible that some human *individuals* exist who lack moral standing (or who lack the moral standing typical of human beings). They do so because, individually, the fail to qualify as rights-bearers. We need to find out whether this is a problem according to this view.

Fukuyama's basic moral outlook

Fukuyama accepts the moral rights view in its hierarchical version. In his criticism of transhumanism, he accepts that having characteristics typical of human beings is sufficient to grant an individual a kind of moral standing, and with moral standing go moral rights. But he fears that superhumans would come to have even stricter moral rights than we have. He also fears the possibility that the technique will be used, at the same time, to create less intelligent beings: humans who are not fully human. These individuals would lack the kind of rights *we* have:

> What will happen to political rights once we are able to, in effect, breed some people with saddles on their backs, and others with boots and spurs? (Fukuyama 2002: 10)

His view of the moral *nature* of transhuman individuals is very gloomy. He seems to believe not only that they would be superior to us, and in possession of special rights, but also that they would carry boots and spurs, i.e., be ruthless, and perceive of themselves as beyond *Gut und Böse*:

> What is ultimately at stake with biotechnology is not just some utilitarian cost-benefit calculus concerning future medical technologies, but the very grounding of the human moral sense, which has been a constant ever since there were human beings. It may be the case that, as Nietzsche predicted, we are fated to move beyond this moral sense. But if so, we

need to accept the consequences of the abandonment of natural standards for right and wrong forthrightly and recognize, as Nietzsche did, that this may lead us into territory that many of us don't want to visit. (Fukuyama 2002: 102)

But what sort of moral theory more precisely does Fukuyama hold? This is what he claims that he is after:

... if we are to find a source of that superior human moral status that raises us all above the rest of animal creation and yet makes us equals of one another qua human beings, we need to know more about that subset of characteristics of human nature that are not just typical of our species but unique to human beings. (Fukuyama 2002: 147)

Now, this may *look* like the idea that humans are special, i.e. it may look like a kind of speciesism. However, appearances are deceptive. On Fukuyama's view, we must qualify individually for human dignity and hence moral standing by exhibiting (among other things) certain *cognitive* capacities, and there is no guarantee that *all* human beings succeed. At least *some* human beings are clearly less human than others. Yet, as a matter of fact, most grown-up human individuals do possess the relevant quality, they do exhibit full human dignity, and are hence entitled to equal political and other legal rights, he claims.

What if it had been otherwise? According to Fukuyama, it is *good* news that there is no conclusive evidence to the effect that some racial groups are superior to others with regard to IQ. He is also confident that such evidence will not be forthcoming:

The amount of evolutionary time that has passed since the races separated is too short, and the degree of genetic variance between the races, when looking at characteristics that can be measured (such as the distribution of blood types), is too narrow to suggest that there can be strong group differences in this regard. (Fukuyama 2002: 31)

Why is this reassuring? I suppose Fukuyama thinks it is reassuring because if the races had differed systematically with regard to IQ (and perhaps some other characteristics as well), then this may have implied that they were not equal with regard to their value and 'dignity', and hence not equal with regard to the political rights they should be given.

But suppose Black Americans had been less intelligent than Asians and Caucasians. If the moral rights theory is *correct*, this means that there *is* a moral difference (with regard to human dignity) between Black Americans on the one hand and Asians and Caucasians on the other hand. But then it would hardly be objectionable if Black Americans were disenfranchised. They have no *moral* right to vote in the first place. Now that we know that there is no such difference, we can safely conclude that Black Americans were wronged in the past when they were disenfranchised. But this is just because, as a matter of fact, they are just as intelligent as Asians,

Caucasians, and other 'racial' groups in the US. Had it been different, they would not have been wronged, on this moral view, when they were disenfranchised.

Moral rights and the argument from nastiness

But perhaps one could argue that a world where there are no such systematic differences with regard to intelligence is *nicer* than a world where such differences exist. This strikes me as a plausible claim. It is not a problem that horses, according to this moral view, have a lower moral standing than (most) human beings. The reason that this is not problematic is that the difference between a human being and a horse is conspicuously clear, and that the horse does not know that he has lower moral standing than a human being. It is different with differences among human beings, if such differences exist. They are in a way nasty. The way in which they are nasty is brought out very clearly in a futurist passage in Fukuyama's book:

> Scientists have not dared to produce a full-scale chimera, half human and half ape, though they could; but young people begin to suspect that class-mates who do much less well than they do are in fact genetically not fully human. Because, in fact, they aren't. (Fukuyama 2002: 9)

Let us pursue this matter a bit further, however. There are groups *other* than the so-called human races that do indeed differ with regard to intelligence. There is in particular a group of people who are *indeed* less intelligent than average human beings. This is true, for example, of the minority group whose members score below 80 on the IQ test. Members of this minority group are *without any exception* less intelligent than most human beings. Does this mean that they are not truly human, and that they do not have a *moral* right to political rights such as the right to vote?

This is hard to tell, on Fukuyama's view, since he is not precise. Being human, in the first place, is to possess a characteristic that *emerges* from an underlying base of more ordinary, mainly cognitive capacities. He speaks of factor X as the factor constituting our full humanity, granting us dignity and equal moral rights, and he claims:

> Factor X cannot be reduced to the possession of moral choice, or reason, or language, or sociability, or sentience, or emotions, or consciousness, or any other quality that has been put forth as a ground for human dignity. It is all of these qualities coming together in a human whole that make up Factor X. (Fukuyama 2002: 171)

I have no problem with the idea that some things emerge from others. I can understand the claim that mental events emerge from physical events, for example

– even if I hold no view on whether this is true or not. I can understand what it means for psychological events to emerge from physical events since I am familiar with psychological events (they happen to me all the time) and since I have some clue about physics. However, the claim that being human (the factor X) emerges from more mundane characteristics is more difficult to assess. I have problems in understanding this claim since I am not familiar with what it means to be human. I am not familiar with the factor X. And yet there seems to be a way of assessing Fukuyama's claim in the present context. We can focus exclusively on one of the relata, the cognitive capacities, in the relation between the base and what emerges from it, Factor X. Which are they? What does it *take* for us to be truly human and to possess dignity and full moral rights?

It is also a good idea to focus on the underlying basis because the use of the term 'human' seems to be a misnomer in Fukuyama's case. There are members of the human species who lack humanity as conceived of by Fukuyama and for all we know there may be members of very different species with which we are not yet familiar who possess humanity.

Fukuyama fears, as we have seen, that we may come to create creatures who are intellectually inferior to us so they can do some hard and dirty work for us. But people with these characteristics already exist! And they often do hard and dirty work for us. So I think Fukuyama should be as concerned about their existence as he is about the possibility that such people will be constructed through genetic engineering.[2]

I get the impression that once you fall below a certain limit on the IQ test, at least if this deficiency is also combined, as it often is, with some kind of emotional and linguistic problems, you are not human in Fukuyama's view. This limit may be, as in my example, 80 on the IQ score, or it may be somewhat lower. However, it seems to be a reasonable conclusion that some people who do not suffer from any disease are yet not fully human, in particular if they score poorly not only in the IQ test but also with regard to the other items on Fukuyama's list, such as linguistic capacity and sociability.

Children typically fail to possess full humanity and dignity in this respect, as Fukuyama notes. Hence we do not grant them political rights such as the right to vote in general elections. Is this an insult to them? Perhaps it is, but first of all we can inform them that this is only fair, since they have not yet developed full dignity and to some extent we can comfort them by pointing out to them that when they grow up, as they will, they *will*, at a certain fixed time, be granted political rights. Something similar is true of people suffering from senile dementia. We do not dis-

---

2.   I concede that if we create people for this purpose we may be adding insult to injury; but in Fukuyama's view their very existence presents us with the problem I discuss, i.e. the problem of nastiness.

enfranchise them, but they cannot use their legal right to vote anyway, and this is as it should be, Fukuyama notes. Like children, they have no moral right to political rights. And even if there is no way we can comfort them – there is indeed no need to do so – at least it is true of them that they have once *been* full human beings. There are other marginal human groups, however, who never mature. They never become, nor have they ever been, full human beings. Hence they lack a moral right to full political rights. I am referring to the people I have just identified: healthy people with low scores on intelligence tests, linguistic tests in particular, and tests for sociability. Is it a problem, according to this view, that they lack full human standing and hence human dignity?

In principle, I suppose it is not a problem. If the moral theory we are currently discussing is correct, then they *have* no right to vote in general elections, for example, so we would not violate their rights if we were to disenfranchise them. And yet I cannot help feeling that if this moral theory had been correct, it would still have been *nicer* if every grown-up human had been fully human. It must be nasty to realise that you have lower moral standing than other individuals who, in many ways, *seem* to be your peers. But if this is true, then biological egalitarianism is what comes to mind. Why not see to it, through positive germ-line genetic engineering, that all (grown-up) human beings *become* fully human? This argument may mean an addition to Fukuyama's view, but it is consistent with what he says and as such very plausible.

As I have indicated, I do not believe in the moral rights theory, so I will not rely on it in any argument in defence of biological (cognitive) egalitarianism. I leave this kind of defence to Fukuyama. Instead I turn to the last approach I will discuss: utilitarianism.

The utilitarian argument

According to utilitarianism, even severely mentally retarded people, and people suffering from senile dementia, as well as many non-human animals, have moral standing. There is no *need* to level up therefore, according to utilitarianism. So could utilitarianism provide us with a rationale not *for* biological egalitarianism, but *against* this idea? The answer is no, and in this section I will show why utilitarian's should actually favour cognitive equality.

If no-one needs to become cleverer in order to obtain moral standing (as I have just argued), and if no-one becomes happier simply by becoming cleverer (which I have argued elsewhere) (Tännsjö 2009: 421-432), then why bother to level up with regard to cognitive capacities?

There seem to be good utilitarian reasons to do so, but they are of an indirect sort.

178

First of all, it seems likely that if a child is provided with a full repertoire of capacities, this renders it easier for the child to embark on the kind of life and career she wants. I recently happened to listen to a person on a bus complaining to a friend that there was one thing he wanted to do, another thing that could bring him a decent income, and a third yet that he knew he was good at. In a world where a person such as this one had all the capacities available for all three possible careers, life would have been easier. In such a world this person might have been less frustrated and hopefully therefore happier.

This argument is, of course, merely speculative. A more substantive argument can be built upon the following observation, however. There are some problematic diseases to which no-one can adapt. I am thinking here in particular of mental illnesses such as depression, anxiety and psychosis. When people suffer from these diseases they do indeed suffer. And we do our best to treat these diseases, or at least to lessen the symptoms. But it would be fine if we could obviate the need for these cures by eliminating the diseases in the first place. This is a controversial claim but a sound claim. It is sometimes said that our world would be less rich without these diseases. This is true. But this is true also of rape, war and torture. Much good literature, for example, is inspired by these phenomena. This does not mean, however, that a world without them, assessed from the point of view of utilitarianism, would be worse than the present world. It would be much better. The 'entertainment' value of phenomena such as these is real, but the suffering of the victims weighs much more heavily in the utilitarian calculus.

Or, should we say that, in a world where no-one suffered from these diseases no art would be produced, since it is crucial that artists suffer from these conditions – otherwise they will not be capable of producing good art? When I read what Fukuyama writes about a world where germ-line genetic enhancement has taken place, I get the impression that this is what he thinks:

> ... it could be the kind of soft tyranny envisioned in *Brave New World*, in which everyone is healthy and happy but has forgotten the meaning of hope, fear, or struggle. (Fukuyama 2002: 218)

Is it true that if we become healthy, we will forget the meaning of hope, fear, or struggle? I don't think so.

Some artists and scientists in the past have suffered from the kind of personality disorders typical of the mental disease we are here discussing. The elimination of these personality disorders is irrelevant at best to their achievements. Often their disease has been detrimental to them, if for no other reason than that it has taken much time and effort from their lives. And even if some of them have occasionally been inspired by their problems, we (humanity) can afford to sacrifice *these* pieces of art – for the sake of the happiness of their creators.

Now, if we were to opt for cognitive equality, these diseases would of course be eliminated. But my claim is stronger. My claim is that personality disorders that cannot easily be described as diseases, such as ADHD and a lack of a capacity for empathy or sociability, should be eliminated as well. And I claim that intelligence should be levelled out (up). Is there a utilitarian rationale for this claim as well?

Yes there is, and it is similar to the rationale behind the need to eliminate certain diseases. Just like diseases, these personality traits create suffering.

In a competitive society, people who lag behind with regard to their cognitive capacities create problems and costs (in terms of well-being) for themselves and others. The most important or at least most obvious example of this is cognitive deficiencies exhibited by healthy people leading to criminal behaviour.

There is a great deal of discussion about the relation between low intelligence and crime, but the correlation is certainly there. There also seems to be a causal mechanism – or many mechanisms, with low intelligence playing a causal role. People with low intelligence are treated worse at school, and hence they often fail in their early education, which makes them prone to criminal behaviour. The lack of cognitive skills, in particular linguistic skills, makes it difficult to develop a capacity to socialise with others. Again, this renders people prone to criminal behaviour. It is true that people with low intelligence are more often caught when they commit crime than people with high intelligence, but that does not seem to suffice to explain away the correlation between low intelligence and criminal behaviour. At least in the kind of highly competitive society where we live, low intelligence tends (together with other causal factors) to produce criminal behaviour (Henry and Moffit 1997: 280-288).

There is also a correlation between a personality disorder called ADHD and crime, which again seems to be causal. Many prisoners all over the world suffer from ADHD, and according to several studies this is no coincidence. It is not only that people with ADHD are more often caught when they commit crime; they commit crime more often than people who do not suffer from this condition. Here is the abstract of one recent and influential study by Jason Fletcher and Barbara Wolfe:

The question of whether childhood mental illness has long-term consequences in terms of criminal behavior has been little studied, yet it could have major consequences for both the individual and society more generally. In this paper, we focus on Attention-Deficit/ Hyperactivity Disorder (ADHD), one of the most prevalent mental conditions in school-age children, to examine the long-term effects of childhood mental illness on criminal activities, controlling for a rich set of individuals, family, and community level variables. The empirical estimates, consistent with economic models of crime that predict that those with less "legal" human capital are more likely to choose to engage in illegal activity, show that children who experience ADHD symptoms face a substantially increased likelihood of engaging in many types of criminal activities. An included "back-of-the-envelope" calculation of the social costs associated with criminal activities by individuals with childhood ADHD finds the costs to be substantial. (Fletcher and Wolfe 2009: abstract).

Crime is detrimental to those who perform criminal actions, i.e. those who become criminals. In particular this is true of those who are caught and punished. Moreover, there are victims of crime, and their suffering also often results in a considerable utilitarian cost. Finally, a system where criminals are put in gaol is extremely costly. If we could reduce the impact of crime on society, this would mean a net gain in happiness. So the utilitarian, indirect argument for cognitive equality, levelling out intelligence at a high level, and eliminating altogether conditions such as ADHD, a psychopathic personality, an antisocial personality, and so forth, to the extent that this is possible, is strong.

What has here been said about ADHD and crime applies in an even more obvious manner to the lack of a capacity for identification with others; not all such conditions are characterised as diseases, yet they are very problematic for those who exhibit them and for others. In some cases part of the explanation why a person has become a criminal is that this person has such a personality trait. When we level out cognitive capacities, we are not only narrowing down the gap between those who are most talented and those who are less talented, we are also helping people who used to be less talented over some critical hurdles; hurdles that are critical, for instance, to a good life in our kind of society.

This does not mean that people with either low intelligence or ADHD, or a lack of a capacity for empathy (psychopaths, sociopaths, and the like), are *destined* to crime or a bad life. There are many mediating causes such as how they are looked upon when young by their teachers, how they are generally taken care of, which kind of opportunities are given them, and so forth, that, together with their special characteristic, do the decisive work. Many of these factors are connected to the fact that we live in a highly competitive society. Indeed they are connected to the fact that advanced societies are becoming *increasingly* competitive and outright meritocratic.

If this is so, it is natural to ask whether we should instead change society? Why should society be so competitive? Could we not, and should we not, relax? After all, there is no need any more, at least for those of us who live in the rich parts of the world, to be so competitive. Should we not change our way of life?

Fine, if we can do it, I would say to this suggestion. But I doubt that this is a feasible political goal. And note that it is probably easier to relax our social ambitions if we live in a biologically equal society rather than in an unequal one. If this is true it constitutes an independent argument for cognitive equality. The argument goes roughly like this.

It is indeed unfair if those who are less talented are paid less than those who are more talented (unless doing so is to the advantage of those who are less talented). We are no more responsible for the tickets we have drawn in the genetic lottery than we are for our 'choice' of parents, as John Rawls has famously pointed out (Rawls 1971: 101[3]). Hence we should level out economic differences. But the fact that this is something we should do does not mean that it is *easy* to level out economic differences in our society. Why it is difficult is explained by Francis Fukuyama in his *empirical* observation that:

> Most people accept the fact that a Mozart or an Einstein or a Michael Jordan has talents and abilities that they don't have, and receives recognition and even monetary compensation for what he accomplishes with those talents. (Fukuyama 2002: 149)

If we all became equals, in particular in our cognitive capacities, there would be no room for *this* kind of lenient view of inequalities. If the reason that some people excel in music and others in mathematics, while others live a quiet life of a more vegetative nature, is that this is what their parents have chosen for them, then we would not be prepared to pay some people more because they are so talented.

There would be room for some economic differences, I suppose, but these differences would be different from the present ones. We would be prepared to pay more to people who work harder or undertake all sorts of dirty business, but not much more than we want to afford ourselves. And, in particular, there would be no way that we can argue that some get more because they are more talented than the rest of us.

There is no denying that today many people believe that there are people who are just meant to do the heavy and dirty work for them, since these people have no talent for anything else. This is a misconception, of course, but there is room for it in a society where people naturally differ with regard to intelligence. In a biologically equal society, where people do not differ (much) with regard to intelligence, there will be no room for it.

The result, I conjecture, if we level out biological differences with regard to our cognitive abilities, would be a more equal and less competitive society, even measured in standard *economic* terms. Furthermore, those who are paid most would be those who deliberately undertake hard and dirty work, not those who are seen as extraordinarily talented. This would be nice. It would also mean a more just society, based on all decent notions of justice. More importantly in the present utilitarian context, this would mean a more *healthy* society too, if we can trust the results published by Richard Wilkinson and Kate Pickett. And they do indeed make a very impressive and convincing statement of their case (Wilkinson and Pickett: 2009).

---

3.   Note that the statement of this position is especially clear in this original edition of the book.

Conclusion

We have seen that a policy of levelling out, in the sense of levelling up, our cognitive capacities, in order to create biological (cognitive) equality – within our species-typical variation – means no threat to our basic moral standing; this is so irrespective of how we assess it, either from the point of view of a speciesist idea according to which humans are special, or from a moral rights theory, or from the point of view of utilitarianism. We have seen, furthermore, that if we want to see to it that our society is nice, in the sense that there is a rationale for granting political rights to at least all adult human beings, the implementation of a policy of cognitive equality gains support from a moral rights theory of the kind advocated by Frances Fukuyama – through what I have referred to as the argument from *nastiness*. It is true that this argument makes no reference to the core of Fukuyama's theory, but it is consistent with it, and it is such that it is highly likely that Fukuyama should welcome it as a reasonable addition to his theory. He would probably accept that when we can make society a better (less nasty) place, without violating any rights, we should do so. Finally, there are very strong indirect utilitarian reasons to level out our cognitive capacities.

The upshot of this is that we can safely conclude that a policy to establish, as soon as it becomes possible, biological (cognitive) equality, is something we should adopt. In particular, genetic germ-line engineering to this effect is a complimentary service a welfare state should offer all its citizens, even if it may seem to them to be an offer they can't refuse.

■ References

Fletcher, Jason and Barbara Wolfe. 2009. 'Long-term Consequences of Childhood ADHD on Criminal Activities', in *The Journal of Mental Health Policy and Economics*, vol. 12: 119-138.

Fukuyama, Francis. 2002. *Our Posthuman Future. Consequences of the Biotechnology* Revolution. New York: Picador.

Henry, B. and T.E. Moffit. 1997. 'Neuropsychologial and neuroimaging studies of juvenile delinquent and adult criminal behaviour', in *Handbook of antisocial behaviour*, eds. D.M. Stoff et al., 280-288. New York: John Wiley & Sons.

Rawls, John. 1971. *A Theory of Justice*. Cambridge, MA: Harvard University Press.

Tännsjö, Torbjörn. 2009. 'Ought We to Enhance Our Cognitive Capacities?', in *Bioethics* vol. 23, no. 7: 421-432.

Tännsjö, Torbjörn. 1993. 'Should We Change the Human Genome?', in *Theoretical Medicine*, vol. 14: 231-247.

Wilkinson, Richard and Kate Pickett. 2009. *The Spirit Level: Why Equality is Better for Everyone*. London: Penguin.

13 Enhancing Equality

Julian Savulescu

The Basic Bioconservative Worry: Inequality

Bioconservatives like Francis Fukuyama, Leon Kass, Michael Sandel, Jurgen Habermas, Bill McKibben and many others worry about enhancement. They see it as threat to human equality and the fundamental dignity of man. This basic worry erupts in the form of various arguments, but the basic concern is, I believe, a unitary one: the Argument from Equality.

Fukuyama puts the worry this way:

> The first victim of transhumanism [the project of enhancing human beings] might be equality. ... Underlying this idea of the equality of rights is the belief that we all possess a human essence that dwarfs manifest differences in skin color, beauty, and even intelligence. This essence, and the view that individuals therefore have inherent value, is at the heart of political liberalism. But modifying that essence is the core of the transhumanist project. If we start transforming ourselves into something superior, what rights will these enhanced creatures claim, and what rights will they possess when compared to those left behind? If some move ahead, can anyone afford not to follow? These questions are troubling enough within rich, developed societies. Add in the implications for citizens of the world's poorest countries for whom biotechnology's marvels likely will be out of reach and the threat to the idea of equality becomes even more menacing. (Fukuyama 2004)

Michael Sandel (2004) argues that by engaging in enhancement we will lose humility, solidarity and a sense of responsibility for the worse off, thereby failing to treat them as equals. Instead, we need to appreciate the "giftedness" of life.

> To appreciate children as gifts is to accept them as they come, not as objects of our design or products of our will or instruments of our ambition. Parental love is not contingent on the talents and attributes a child happens to have. .... Their qualities are unpredictable, and even the most conscientious parents cannot be held wholly responsible for the kind of children they have. That is why parenthood, more than other human relationships, teaches what the theologian William F. May calls an 'openness to the unbidden.' May's resonant phrase helps us see that the deepest moral objection to enhancement lies ... in the hubris of the

designing parents, in their drive to master the mystery of birth. Even if this disposition did not make parents tyrants to their children, it would disfigure the relation between parent and child, and deprive the parent of the humility and enlarged human sympathies that an openness to the unbidden can cultivate. (Michael Sandel)

Being open to the unbidden is important, for Sandel, in fostering humility, responsibility and solidarity.

A lively sense of the contingency of our gifts – a consciousness that none of us is wholly responsible for his or her success – saves a meritocratic society from sliding into the smug assumption that the rich are rich because they are more deserving than the poor... (Michael Sandel).

It is obvious, even to bioconservatives, that we are all born unequal. Some have wretched diseases from birth and die young. Others abuse their bodies for a lifetime, yet live long. Some are strong, others are weak. Some are beautiful, others are ugly. Some are stupid, others are smart. It is not often put as bluntly as that, but most of us know that no two people, even identical twins, are identical, and nor are they exactly equal in any physical, psychological or social state.

However, equality as a moral ideal is not a description of the way the world is or how people are, but an ideal of how people should be treated: that regardless of these existing physical, psychological and social inequalities, they should be treated equally as persons (Singer 1985). This can mean many things, but the core idea is that by virtue of his or her humanity, each person has an entitlement to be considered in the same way as any other person. So each person's suffering, hunger, thirst and other basic needs matter equally. The life of each person matters equally and should be treated by political institutions, the law and social norms equally.

Bioconservatives worry that either the motivation to enhance, the act of enhancement or the result of enhancement will constitute inequality or lead to people being treated unequally. How could this be so? Since equality is a prescriptive ideal, how could changing the empirical world affect the nature of, or the effectiveness of, a moral prescription? Since these are different ontological categories, it is puzzling how these writers relate one to the other. The problematic nature of this relationship can be seen through an analogy.

Imagine that I am a caterer running a children's party. I bring out the birthday cake. I am told to divide it equally amongst the 10 children. According to the Objection from Equality, something I do to the children may affect my equal division of the cake. How could modification of the 10 children affect my division? Well, if I had given one of the children plenty of food already, that child would not be hungry. If I hypnotized a child to have an aversion to cake, that child would not want the cake. If I had invited one of my own children, I might want to give that child a bigger slice.

But notice that none of these modifications necessarily leads to me divide the cake unequally. Nor does it affect the truth of the fact, if it is indeed a truth, that the cake should be divided equally. It is up to me to divide the cake into 10 equal pieces or not. The children might react differently to receiving their piece, or I might feel differently about it, but they would still receive an equal share if I respected equality.

The proponents of the Objection from Equality engage in aversion of the naturalistic fallacy. While they do not derive an "is" from an "ought", but they do that "is" affects or somehow determines or changes "ought". "Ought" might imply "can" but it does not imply "is". If I ought to divide the cake equally, this is not affected merely by contingent empirical facts, such as my feelings, the children's feelings, or whether they have been enhanced or not. What I ought to do is determined by certain normative facts or principles, together with relevant empirical facts.

Perhaps the bioconservative worry is a more pragmatic one. Perhaps they worry that the way the world is and the way people are, various enhancements *will* lead to people being unethically treated more unequally. This is a pure empirical speculation without any robust evidence adduced to support it.

Here is one way in which it seems unlikely. Consider two children: one of them is a gifted musician by nature, while the other has been enhanced to be a gifted musician. The first does not owe her success to anyone. She was just lucky. Those who win a lottery do not feel a debt to the other losers who are now worse off than them. By contrast, the enhanced musician owes a debt to the person who enhanced her. Indeed, Habermas worries that this relationship is so strong that the enhanced is subordinated to the will of the enhancer.

Sandel's worry can be turned on its head. If the enhancer is the State, the enhanced owes a debt to the State (to the people who contributed to and made possible her enhancement). This would increase a sense of solidarity and fellow concern.

However, I will now give two other arguments that enhancement would reduce rather than increase inequality. The first addresses the brute fact that natural inequality exists with profound consequences for how individuals' lives develop, the quality of their relationships and morality. Enhancement can be used to correct this natural inequality. Secondly, the concern that individuals will care less about others and will be more disposed to treat others unjustly can be addressed by enhancing the very mechanisms involved in these dispositions. That is, we can enhance the moral dispositions that cause social inequality.

What is Justice?

There are several theories of justice, including Utilitarianism, Egalitarianism, and Prioritarianism (this section on Justice is drawn from Savulescu 2009: 177-187).

Utilitarians argue that enhancements should be distributed to provide the greatest benefits to the greatest number (i.e. to bring about the most good). Enhancement is not unjust if some people are worse off, even badly off, provided that enhancements are distributed according to a principle of equality that holds that each individual should count for one and that nobody should count for more than one. That is, provided that enhancements are allocated strictly to bring about the greatest good, with no eye to social privilege, status, wealth or other irrelevant consideration, then that distribution is just.

Egalitarians argue that enhancements should be distributed so as to provide equal consideration of equal needs. Enhancements should alleviate need in individuals as much as possible. The greater a person's need, the greater that person's entitlement to resources. According to one egalitarian theory of justice, Rawls' Justice as Fairness, we should distribute enhancements so that the worst off in society are as well off as they can be (Rawls 1971). According to Prioritarians (Parfit 1997: 202-221), we should not give absolute priority to the worst off, it does give some priority to those who are worst off, but we should also aim to maximise the well-being of all members of society.

In "Rights, Utility and Universalization" (Mackie 1984: 86-105), John Mackie suggests that everyone has a 'right to a fair go'. According to a maximizing version of giving people a "fair go," we should give as many people as possible a decent (reasonable) chance of having a decent (good) life. This is a plausible common-sense principle of justice which has also been called "sufficientarianism".

I find "a fair go" to be a plausible conception of justice. Getting a "fair go" means having a fair chance of receiving an intervention that has a reasonable chance of providing a reasonable extension of one's life and/or a reasonable improvement in its quality, or access to basic goods necessary for those. A fair go entails that each person has a legitimate claim to medical care when that care provides that person with a reasonable chance of reasonable extension of a reasonable life and/or a reasonable improvement in its quality. Comparable legitimate claims are those referring to similar needs. As many comparable legitimate claims should be satisfied as possible. Provided as many comparable legitimate claims are being satisfied as possible, there should be equality of access.

However, for the present argument, which substantive view of justice we accept does not matter. For the purposes of argument, I will adopt the right to a fair go. However, any of the other accounts of justice could be used to make similar points.

The Profound Consequences of Natural Biopsychological Inequality[1]

■ Well-Being

Many biological and psychological characteristics can profoundly affect how well our lives progress and whether we have a "fair go". One example is impulse control. In the 1960s Walter Mischel conducted impulse control experiments in which 4-year-old children were left in a room with one marshmallow each, after being told that if they did not eat the marshmallow, they could later have two. Some children ate it as soon as the researcher left, while others used a variety of strategies to help control their behaviour and ignore the temptation of the single marshmallow. A decade later, the researchers re-interviewed the children and found that those who were better at delaying gratification had more friends, better academic performance and more motivation to succeed. Whether the child had grabbed for the marshmallow had a much stronger bearing on their SAT scores (the USA's standardised test for college admissions) than did their IQ (Mischel et al. 1988). Impulse control has also been linked to socioeconomic control and avoiding conflict with the law.

Impulse control is what some philosophers call an "All Purpose Good": it is a good for a person no matter what that person's plan for life or particular way of being or context. Self-control is valuable whether you want to be a philosopher, doctor, builder, entertainer or soldier. Other examples of all purpose goods include memory, self-discipline, foresight, patience, a sense of humour, and optimism.

■ Cognitive Inequality[2]

One of the most important all purpose goods is general intelligence, or g (short for the $g$eneral mental ability factor). This is a proficiency in learning, reasoning and thinking abstractly. It is the ability to spot problems and to solve them. It is not specific knowledge, but the ability to accumulate and apply it.

General intelligence or g naturally varies in a normal distribution within a given, defined population. For western populations, it famously follows a bell curve with a mean of 100 and a standard deviation of 15 points. Intellectual disability for medical, legal and social purposes is arbitrarily defined as an IQ two standard deviations below the mean (below 70). However, where one finds oneself on this curve as a result of the natural lottery profoundly affects one's life chances and opportunities, what one can do and who one can be.

---

1. This section on the Consequences of Natural Inequality is drawn from Savulescu (2010).
2. I would like to thank Prof. Linda Gottfredson for valuable data and for opening my eyes to the social implications of intelligence. See http://www.udel.edu/educ/gottfredson for a full archive of her groundbreaking work.

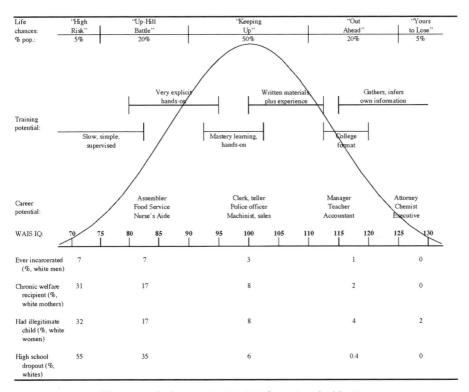

Life chances:	"High Risk"	"Up-Hill Battle"	"Keeping Up"	"Out Ahead"	"Yours to Lose"
% pop.:	5%	20%	50%	20%	5%

Training potential: Very explicit, hands-on | Written materials plus experience | Gathers, infers own information

Slow, simple, supervised | Mastery learning, hands-on | College format

| Career potential: | | Assembler Food Service Nurse's Aide | Clerk, teller Police officer Machinist, sales | Manager Teacher Accountant | Attorney Chemist Executive |

WAIS IQ: 70 75 80 85 90 95 100 105 110 115 120 125 130

Ever incarcerated (%, white men)	7	7	3	1	0
Chronic welfare recipient (%, white mothers)	31	17	8	2	0
Had illegitimate child (%, white women)	32	17	8	4	2
High school dropout (%, whites)	55	35	6	0.4	0

Figure 1. Source of figure: Gottfredson, 1997: 79-132, figure 3 and table 10.

For example, the US Department of Education (1993) estimated the levels of typical cognitive functioning of American adults in its National Adult Literacy Survey (NALS). This involved a nationally representative sample of 26,000 individuals aged 16-65. It grouped scores into five levels of functioning. The following table illustrates these levels of functioning, together with the fraction of adults for whom this is the maximum level of functioning they achieve in everyday tasks.

The US Department of Education has stated that people at Levels 1-2 are below the literacy level required for "competing successfully in a global economy and exercising fully the rights and responsibilities of citizenship" (Baldwin, et al. 1995; Gottfredson 1997: 114).

The US Army has long known that people with intelligence at the low end of the normal range are unfit intellectually for military service. The army administers IQ-like tests of "trainability". Since the second world war, the army has been forbidden by law from inducting anyone from the bottom 10% (IQ 80 and below), and its own minimum standards rule out anyone below the 15th percentile (below IQ 85). In practice, entry into most military jobs requires scores above the 30th percentile (above IQ

189

Figure 2.

NALS Level	% pop.	Simulated Everyday Tasks
5	3%	• Use calculator to determine cost of carpet for a room • Use table of information to compare 2 credit cards
4	17%	• Use eligibility pamphlet to calculate SSI benefits • Explain difference between 2 types of employee benefits
3	31%	• Calculate miles per gallon from mileage record chart • Write brief letter explaining error on credit card bill
2	27%	• Determine difference in price between 2 show tickets • Locate intersection on street map
1	22%	• Total bank deposit entry • Locate expiration date on driver's license

92), which means that about a third of induction-age youth lack the cognitive ability to qualify for even the simplest jobs in the army (Gottfredson 1998).

The lowest level involves being able to perform tasks no more difficult than totalling two entries on a bank deposit slip or locating the expiration date on a driving licence. For 22% of Americans, this is the highest level of functioning which they can achieve with 80% probability. Level 2 tasks are more cognitively complex because they require the use of two pieces of information, drawing a simple inference and ignoring a bit of distracting information. An example of this is determining the difference in price between two show tickets listed on a simple flyer or locating a specific intersection on a street map. For 27% of Americans, this is the highest level of functioning; they cannot routinely do more complicated tasks, such as calculating miles per gallon from a mileage record chart – a Level 3 task. NALS Level 2 corresponds roughly to IQs of 86-97 (Gottfredson: 1997).

The US Army is not constrained by political correctness or fine-sounding ideological redescriptions of reality. One representative from the Defence Advanced Research Projects Agency wrote: "The world contains approximately 4.2 billion people over the age of twenty. Even a small enhancement of cognitive capacity in these individuals would probably have an impact on the world economy rivalling that of the internet".[3]

Cognitive Enhancement is one way of overcoming one of the biological barriers to a good life and a life of opportunity. And it can be cheap. One in three people in the world don't get enough iodine. This can cause mental slowness. A deficiency of iodine in pregnancy results in the loss of 10 to 15 IQ points in the fetus. Around the world, this results in more than 1 billion IQ points of mental capital being lost each year. Iodising salt costs only two to three cents per person per year. There may

---

3.   See US Army: Proposal Submission, at http://www.dodsbir.net/solicitation/sttr08A/army08A.htm.

be other cheap methods of cognitive enhancement. For example, choline (which occurs naturally in eggs) may increase fetal IQ if given in pregnancy.

As drugs are developed to treat memory loss in Alzheimer's disease, these drugs are likely to be effective also for normal age-related memory loss, which occurs after the age of 40.

Drugs are already being used to improve cognitive performance in the normal range. Modafinil is a new class of drug originally developed for narcolepsy. It is now also prescribed for shift workers. It improves executive function, wakefulness, and working memory. It is now widely used by academics, other professionals and college students in the US to enhance cognitive performance. Used daily it would cost about $100-$200 per month, compared to smoking one pack of cigarettes per day, which costs $60 per month.

It has been estimated that "Ninety percent of the prescriptions are for off-label usage".[4] Sales of this drug have grown exponentially. One version, Provigil (Cephalon), has increased sales from $75 million in 2001 to $500 million in 2005. If this growth were to continue, the market in 2018 would be $US70 billion. Modafinil will go generic in 2012, which will mean it will probably only be worth US$7-10 billion in 10 years' time.

In April 2008, an online survey of individuals who read the journal *Nature* revealed that roughly one in five respondents use prescription drugs to improve their focus, concentration or memory (Maher, 2008). A total of 1,400 people from 60 countries responded to the online survey. The subjects were asked specifically about the use of three drugs. Here are the fractions of respondents who had used them:

1. Methylphenidate (Ritalin) 62%
2. Modafinil (Provigil) 44%
3. Beta-blockers 15%

Other drugs were also used:

- Adderall, a drug prescribed for ADHD containing a mixture of amphetamines
- Centrophenoxine
- Piracetam
- Dextroamphetamine Sulfate
- Ginkgo
- Omega-3 fatty acids.

---

4. See http://www.provigilweb.org/p12.htm.

Figure 3.

Drug	Effect	+	-
Sugar	Stimulates, memory improvement, self-control improvement	Legal, very cheap, safe, well studied	Bad for teeth
Modafinil	Increased alertness, better executive function	Well studied, apparently safe and non-addictive	Risk of overexertion?
Caffeine	Increased alertness	Legal, very cheap, safe, well studied	Quasi-addictive
Nicotine (enhancing cholinergic drugs)	Increased alertness, memory enhancement	Legal	Biased studies? Addictive, smoking unhealthy
Choline	Enhance memory in offspring of pregnant rats	Easily accessible, legal, long-term effects	Unknown long-term side effects
Amphetamine	Increased alertness, memory enhancement, reorganisation	Well studied	Not legal, addictive, preservation
Dopaminergic drugs (e.g. Ritalin)	Attention, working memory		Recreational use
Beta blockers	Calming, reduce impact of anxiety in traumatic memory		
Ampakines	Memory enhancement, increased alertness		Experimental, seizure risk?
CREB-inhibitors	Memory enhancement		Experimental

There are a range of other enhancers available even today.

Cognitive enhancers could be used to correct natural inequality and give people a "fair go". If we used cognitive enhancers to bring as many people as possible above the line of sufficient cognitive functioning, we would be both correcting natural inequality and promoting justice. Where does this line lie? It certainly does not lie at an IQ of 70, where the line is currently arbitrarily drawn. The US Department of Education has stated that people at Levels 1-2 are below the literacy level required for "competing successfully in a global economy and exercising fully the rights and responsibilities of citizenship". The upper limit of Level 2 corresponds to an IQ of about 97. So for practical purposes, we could aim to increase the cognitive abilities of the bottom half of the population: all those with an IQ less than 100. None of this implies that these cognitive limitations are primarily biological (though their causation is likely a mixture of biology and sociological). It is important to recognise that embracing biological enhancement does not imply biological causation. There is nothing intrinsically wrong with employing biological solutions to social problems.

What we want is the best solution to the problem, and that might be biological or biological/social. The differences in IQ might be entirely due to social inequality, although I strongly doubt that this is the case. However, given the way the world is, the best solution might still be some kind of biologically assisted, enhanced education programme (Savulescu 2010).

■ Natural Biopsychological Inequality and Moral Behaviour

Not only does our own biology and psychology limit our cognitive performance, with profound consequences even for normal people in some cases. It can also represent a constraint on us acting morally.

An extreme example is psychopathy. In 1993 two bodies were found on a country road in Ellis County, Texas. One was male, one female. The boy, 14, had been shot, but the 13-year-old girl had been stripped, raped, and dismembered. Her head and hands were missing. They were killed by Jason Massey, aged 20. He was a psychopath.

Massey was nine years old when he killed his first cat. He added dozens more over the years, along with dogs and even six cows. He had a long list of potential victims and his diaries were filled with fantasies of rape, torture, and cannibalism of female victims. He was a loner who believed he served a "master" who gave him knowledge and power. He was obsessed with bringing girls under his control and having their dead bodies in his possession.

We are all familiar with stories about psychopaths. Such people seem to profoundly lack normal human empathy. Often, even their parents realise there is something wrong with them, even from a very young age.

> I have had to work so very hard to distance myself emotionally from my own daughter. I would do anything to make it 'right'. My husband and I have done everything in our power to help her. We can do no more. I still love her, but I know that she is who she is, and that just about kills me. (Narcissist Personality Disorder Forum 2011)

> I also have a son 18 years of age. He has exhibited problems since childhood. He also has rages, lies. Manipulates. He is now off to a very good college and is extremely bright, which actually makes it more lethal. He just hasn't been right since birth. He is no longer living with me and I pray he does well in life. My therapist said I did everything I possibly could for him including therapy since age 3. (Narcissist Personality Disorder Forum 2011)

According to the major textbook of psychiatry (*DSM-III-R* 1987: 343-344):

> Antisocial Personality Disorder is five times more common among first-degree biological relatives of males with the disorder than among the general population. The risk to first-degree biologic relatives of females with the disorder is nearly ten times that of the general

population...Adoption studies show that both genetic and environmental factors contribute to the risk of this group of disorders, because parents with Antisocial Personality Disorder increase the risk of Antisocial Personality Disorder... in both their adopted and biologic children.

In other words, there are good reasons to believe that antisocial personality disorder and psychopathic behaviour have significant biological and even genetic contributors.

People with an antisocial personality have a limited range of human emotions, and in particular they lack empathy for the suffering of others. Empathy may be provided by some remarkable neurons located in the inferior frontal cortex and the anterior part of the inferior parietal lobule of the brain. These nerve cells are active when specific actions such as picking an object of food and eating are performed; but what makes them remarkable is that they also fire when another animal, the experimenter or even a robot performs the same action. A mirror neuron fires as though the observer were performing the action. Evidence is mounting that the region of the brain known as the insula provides the substrate for our understanding of the emotions of others.

The activity of insula neurons underpins the emotion of disgust. The mirror system for hand actions and the mirror system for emotions are more active in people who are empathic as judged by questionnaires. The same thing applies to children, in whom the degree of activity of mirror neurons induced by observations and imitation of facial expression correlated with empathic concern and interpersonal competence. Children with autism-spectrum disorders who are socially isolated and have difficulty demonstrating warmth and interpersonal connectivity also have disturbed activation of the mirror neurons. There are good reasons to believe that autism-spectrum disorders have a strong genetic causation. So at least in these groups, not only is there an emerging biological pathway being identified, but the ultimate cause of such behaviour may be strongly genetically influenced.

Mirror neurons are thus important candidates to represent what philosophers call the "Theory of Mind", or the ability to infer other people's mental states, thoughts and feelings.

The upshot of this is that our own biology and psychology may represent barriers preventing us from empathising with other people and from understanding their mental states. At any rate, there is the prospect that biopsychological interventions could enhance moral behaviour. A crude example of this is the chemical castration of paedophiles. Here, the use of hormonal manipulation to reduce sex drive is offered to paedophiles to reduce the frequency of re-offending.

Psychopathy is not the only example of failed moral behaviour. Ordinary criminal behaviour is another example, and this too may be influenced by biology. Caspi and colleagues investigated the relationship between the presence of a change in the gene encoding for monoamine oxidase A (MAOA), a neurotransmitter metabolising enzyme, and the tendency towards antisocial behaviour in a large cohort of New Zealand males (Capsi et al. 2002). They found that men who had been mistreated as children *and* were positive for the polymorphism conferring low levels of MAOA were significantly more likely to exhibit antisocial behaviour than those who had been mistreated but lacked the change. Both groups were more likely to exhibit antisocial behaviour than those who were not mistreated. This suggests a possible interaction between mistreatment and MAOA deficiency in causing antisocial behaviour. It also raises the possibility that the pharmacological manipulation of MAOA may influence the development of such behaviour.

The neurotransmitter serotonin has been linked to less aggressive behaviour. There is an inverse relationship between indices of serotenergic function and impulsive aggressive behaviour. For example, depleting serotonin leads to more aggressive behaviour. And drugs such as Selective Serotonin Reuptake Inhibitors like Prozac increase cooperation and reduce aggression. Perhaps violent offenders should be on Prozac! At least, we should study its effect scientifically.

Oxytocin, a hormone released by the hypothalamus, has been shown to influence the ability to infer another person's mental state. It increases our willingness to trust other people, but this does not extend to all risk-taking, only to social risks. For example, it prevents the decrease of trust after betrayal, even after several betrayals. It also reduces the fear of social betrayal.

The degree to which we are prepared to trust others and are willing to cooperate, especially in large groups, varies from one individual to the next. This variation has a biological basis that can be altered by biological interventions. For example, by the administration of oxytocin and drugs like Prozac.

None of these interventions represents pure or effective "moral enhancers". But the science of moral enhancement is perhaps like the science of cancer 100 years ago. We have yet to scratch the surface. Yet these show that biologically influencing moral behaviour is possible in principle.

It is important to recognize that important moral failing is not restricted to criminals. All of us fail morally in important ways. In a series of 6 publications with Ingmar Persson[5], we have argued that ordinary people have moral dispositions which are limited in important ways by virtue of our evolutionary history. We have limited altruism, restricted to small in-groups, we tend to free ride, derogate members of out-groups, are biased towards the near future, not prone to make significant sacrifices, and our ordinary morality has evolved to have strong proscrip-

---

5. http://bit.ly/egA9aF.

tions against harming in-group members but no requirements to aid, especially to aid out-group members. In addition, we believe that there is a moral difference between the consequences of what we intentionally do and what we foreseeably and avoidably allow to occur. These features of ourselves, we have argued, make solving global collective action problems like climate change and global poverty very difficult to address through voluntary action.

Even our conceptions of fairness may be determined in part by our own individual biopsychological natures. Here is one reason to believe this. In the Ultimatum Game, there are two players, a proposer and a responder. The proposer divides a reward. For example, the proposer can divide 10 rewards between two pots in different ways (five and five or eight and two, for instance). The proposer can choose one of two trays, each with two pots with a different distribution of rewards. The responder then accepts his share or can reject the offer altogether, in which case each gets nothing.

When this experiment is done with chimps, responders generally accepted 2/8 distributions without any sign of dissatisfaction, even when there was an equal distribution of five raisins in each pot on the alternative tray. In contrast, under similar conditions, adult human responders as a rule respond by rejecting the offer, thereby forgoing a smaller reward in order to punish the proposers for their blatant unfairness.

However, humans differ in terms of how much unfairness they will tolerate in the Ultimatum Game. Some will accept a 4/6 distribution; others only 5/5. What is remarkable is not that humans differ from each other, but that when human identical twins play the proposer and responder roles of the Ultimatum Game, there is a striking correlation between the average division with respect to both what they propose and what they are ready to accept as responders. There is no such correlation in the case of fraternal twins. Since identical twins share the same genes (and these twins have been separated at birth), this strongly suggests that the human sense of fairness has some genetic basis. In humans, the rejection of unfair offers is more than 40% genetically determined, with a very modest role for environmental influences.

In the body of work cited above, Persson and I have argued that we should embrace the possibility that the modification of our moral dispositions by pharmacological and other biological manipulation should be considered and explored. Such an argument addresses the concerns of bioconservatives regarding inequality. Our moral dispositions and choices create social inequality. One way to address that inequality is to change the dispositions of people who make those choices. After all, gross social inequality already exists. It is time to treat the cause rather than the symptom of the disease. And the disease is our limited set of moral dispositions.

■ Biopsychological Inequality and Autonomy

Another familiar objection to enhancement employed by Jürgen Habermas is that when parents choose to enhance their children, they are subjecting the individual to the will of somebody else. Sometimes this is put in terms of a child's right to an open future, based on the idea that children should be left in their natural state until they are competent to decide whether and how to change.

This objection fails for two reasons. Firstly, in many cases there is no maximally open future but different mutually exclusive futures. An example is gender assignment for intersex conditions. For many years, children born with ambiguous genitalia were assigned to be female, and surgically modified to appear fully female. The argument was that it was important for parents to bond and parents needed a certain sex. And it was important to shield the child from the cruel teasing and social discrimination that an uncertain sex would invite. However, many people with intersex conditions now resent the modifications made to them. They wish they had been given the choice to remain as they were born, or to decide themselves which sex they wanted to be once they had grown into adulthood.

This might be regarded as a straightforward case where options should be left open, with the open future argument implying that sex should not be assigned. But this is false. The choice is between two mutually exclusive lives: one involving early sex assignment and (supposedly) greater bonding and higher self esteem, and the other involving an open sexual assignment but greater teasing and lower self esteem. I am not arguing in favour of sex assignment. I am arguing that parents and doctors are faced with two options with different risks and benefits.

To take another example: being a great musician requires training from a very early age. One cannot leave the enhancement of musical talent until a child is grown up, because then it will be too late. If it is employed, such enhancement must be employed early if it is going to be effective.

These arguments about the compromise of autonomy fail for a more important reason related to natural inequality. Autonomy is not merely competent choice. It is rational choice. I have argued for this claim at length (Savulescu 1994, 1995, 1997, 2007; Savulescu and Momeyer 1997), but here is a synopsis. Autonomy is self-determination. It involves self-understanding and forming a conception of what life is best for oneself. It involves evaluating options according to their consequences and how likely those consequences are, and how those consequences match one's own evaluative judgements for one's own life. Mere choice is what characterises animal behaviour. Autonomous choice is normatively evaluative choice.

Now plainly autonomy requires rationality on such an account. But rationality is not equally distributed: people vary in terms of their rationality, and even within the same individual rationality varies from time to time, being influenced by a whole host of situational and contextual circumstances.

Since Kahneman and Tversky first began to describe the psychological biases and heuristics that constrain human rationality, increasing numbers of psychological barriers to fully rational decision-making, even means-end rationality, have been identified. But increasingly we are also coming to understand how states of our own biology can frustrate rational choice and how it might be manipulated to improve rationality and so enhance autonomy.

In recent work from Cambridge, Coates and colleagues described how levels of testosterone and cortisol (naturally occurring hormones) could lead to irrational decision-making, which could in turn contribute to financial crisis (Coates & Herbert 2008). This is not to say that hormonal fluctuations have caused recent financial crises; but they may well have contributed. While their focus was on financial decisions, their findings have implications for how autonomous decisions are when they are influenced by hormonal factors.

Coates and colleagues found that city traders who have high morning testosterone levels make more than average profits for the rest of that day. These researchers hypothesised that this may be because testosterone has been found to increase confidence and the appetite for risk – qualities that would augment the performance of any trader who had a positive expected return. However, previous studies have shown that administered testosterone can lead to irrational decision-making. So if testosterone continued to rise or became chronically elevated, it could begin to have the opposite effect on a trader's profitability by increasing risk-taking to unprofitable levels. They argued that this is because testosterone has also been found to lead to impulsivity and sensation-seeking, to harmful risk taking, and in extreme cases (such as among users of anabolic steroids) to euphoria and mania.

Testosterone may therefore underlie a secondary consequence of the 'winner effect' in which a previous win in the markets leads to increased, and eventually irrational risk-taking in the next round of trading.

Professor Joe Herbert, from the Cambridge Centre for Brain Repair, has said:

> Market traders, like some other occupations (such as air traffic controllers), work under extreme pressure and the consequences of the rapid decisions they have to make can have profound consequences for them, and for the market as a whole. Our work suggests that these decisions may be biased by emotional and hormonal factors that have not so far been considered in any detail ... (Coates and Herbert 2008)[6]

I described before the importance of impulse control and the ability to delay gratification. If one is not able to withstand temptation it is impossible to set and achieve long term goals for one's own life. A person incapable of standing back, of rationally

---

6. http://www.sciencedaily.com/releases/2008/04/080414174855.htm.

reflecting, would not be an autonomous agent. He would be an animal. The degree to which this is possible varies from person to person, and is open to enhancement.

■ Inequality and Love

There are a number of biopsychological constraints on our capacity to love which are a product of our evolution (Savulescu & Sandberg 2007). And these are distributed unequally across humans.

Love for humans, as other animals, passes through three stages:

1. *Lust* promotes mating with any appropriate partner.
2. *Attraction* makes us choose and prefer a particular partner.
3. *Attachment* allows pairs to cooperate and stay together until their parental duties have been completed.

Each of these states has a different basis in brain activity associated with the activation of different neurotransmitters and hormones. Neuroimaging of studies of romantic love has shown activations in regions linked to the oxytocin and vasopressin systems, activation in reward systems, and systematic deactivation in regions linked to negative affect, social judgement and the assessment of other people's emotions and intentions.

For various reasons, including evolutionary considerations, each of these states may pass or disappear. And this is amenable to biological manipulation. Consider the example of attachment, which is involved in pair bonding. The failure of pair bonding is part of the explanation for increasing divorce rates, which are approaching 50% of marriages in many countries.

Much work in social neuroscience studying pair bonding has gone into examining the mating habits of monogamous prairie voles (*Microtus ochrogaster*) and closely related but polygamous meadow voles (*M. montanus*) (e.g. Winslow et al. 1993; Young et al. 1999; Lim et al. 2004). The vole pair bonding systems are based on the neurohormones oxytocin and vasopressin. These also modulate other social interactions such as infant-parent attachment and social recognition and trust. The receptors for these hormones are distributed differently in monogamous and polygamous voles.

The sexual behaviour of these voles can be altered. The infusion of oxytocin into the brains of female prairie voles and vasopressin in male prairie voles facilitated pair bonding even in the absence of mating (while the non-monogamous meadow voles were unaffected). Researchers used gene therapy to introduce a gene from the monogamous male prairie vole into the brain of the closely related but polygamous meadow vole. Genetically modified meadow voles became monogamous, behaving like prairie voles. This gene, which controls a part of the brain's reward centre, is known as the vasopressin receptor gene.

A recent study identified a similar gene in humans: the Vasopressin Receptor 1a (AVPRIA) gene (Walum et al. 2008). This has previously been associated with autism, age at first sexual intercourse, altruism, and creative dance performance. This study assessed relationships on a Pair Bonding Scale (PBS) and found pair bonding was significantly lower for men carrying allele (gene variant) 334 than for those who did not have this allele. The effect was dose dependent – pair bonding was even lower for carriers of 2×334 alleles.

What this shows is that people are not equally fit for certain kinds of relationships. Carriers of the 334 variant more often reported marital crisis, including the threat of divorce in the last year. 15% of men with no 334 allele reported such a crisis, compared to 34% of men with two copies. The frequency of unmarried men was higher among 2 x allele 334 carriers (32%) than men with no 334 allele (17%), even though all the cohabiting individuals in the trial had been in a relationship for at least five years and the majority of all the couples involved were the biological parents of adolescent children. Women also expressed more dissatisfaction with partners who carried the 334 allele: women married to men with 1 or 2 x allele 334 reported lower affection expression, dyadic consensus and dyadic cohesion. The 334 variant is associated with increased activation of the amygdala, which is a brain region known to be of importance for pair bonding. These findings suggest that people may vary in their capacity to sustain a long-term loving relationship. This capacity is amenable to alteration.

Radical Possibilities

Drugs like Modafinil and Ritalin scratch at the surface of enhancing human capacities and increasing human freedom by removing biological and psychological limitations on human freedom to act and be. But more radical modifications are possible in principle. Scientists have created a range of radically enhanced non-human animals. The most striking example is Supermouse, created by scientists at Case Western Reserve University in Cleveland, Ohio. Supermouse is a genetically engineered mouse which runs for up to six hours at a speed of 20 metres per minute before needing a rest. This results from changes to the metabolism of glucose. The genetic change means that the glucose metabolising gene – PEPCK-C – is over-expressed in the skeletal muscle, which avoids the muscle-cramping effects of build-up of lactic acid, which is normally experienced during prolonged exercise. The researchers will use the new mouse to study the effects of diet and exercise on longevity and cancer risk, and potentially to better understand the genetic basis of inherited conditions that lead to muscle wasting in humans.

Supermouse is more active: it has seven times more cage activity than normal mice. It has greater endurance – it ran 6 km on a treadmill (compared with the normal mouse, who could only manage 0.2 km). It has improved metabolism – it ate 60% more but had half the body weight and only 10% of the body fat of a normal mouse. It had an extended lifespan: 'survived longer and looked healthier'. It had extended youthfulness: mice of 30 months were still twice as fast as six-month-old normal mice and were reproductively active at 21 months (and up to 30 months), which is equivalent to being reproductively active as a woman at the age of 80. Supermouse was healthier and had lower cholesterol levels.

Humans have the same gene as supermouse. We could create superhumans today with the same abilities as supermouse. Scientists have recently created a fluorescent human embryo by successfully transferring a gene from a jellyfish into a human embryo. This proves in principle what has long been known in non-human animals. Transferring genes from one species to another can be safe and effective, as can genetic engineering.

At present, scientists are trying to unravel the genetic contribution to human physical and mental ability, performance and behaviour in the field of behavioural genetics. For example, scientists are trying to elucidate the contribution of differences in genetics to aggression and criminal behaviour, alcoholism and addiction, anxiety, personality disorders, psychiatric diseases, homosexuality, maternal behaviour, memory and intelligence, personality traits such as neuroticism and novelty seeking, and sprint/endurance performance in sport. This knowledge may make it possible to predict behaviour and ability, as well as opening the door to biological interventions to improve performance. But as animal research has shown, it is clearly possible in principle to radically improve performance.

Conclusion

Our biological and psychological nature as individuals represents a barrier to our own well-being, to moral behaviour and to love. And these barriers are unequally distributed. Far from being a threat to equality, enhancement may be required for people to be treated equally. This is true in two ways. If employed according to a principle of justice, like sufficientarianism to provide as many people as possible with a fair go, enhancements could be used to correct natural inequality in cognitive ability, moral disposition, capacity to love and autonomy. Secondly and most importantly, they could be used to enhance the very dispositions which create social inequality. Our sense of fairness, empathy, sympathy, willingness to make self-sacrifices, commitment to equality vary naturally from individual; they are influenced by biological factors; we could use biology to enhance the attitudes and commitments to achieve equality.

There are four ways to increase equality. We can do so by altering our natural environment, social environment, psychology and biology. We should consider *all* options and make an active, reasoned choice. We should not privilege biological or psychological interventions over social change, but should consider them all as candidates for improvement.

If equality is an ideal worth achieving, I strongly suspect we will have to change the dispositions of people to achieve it.

■ References

Baldwin, J. et al. 1995. *The literacy proficiencies of GED examinees: Results from the GED-NALS comparison study*. Washington D.C.: American Council on Education and Educational Testing. Quoted in Gottfredson, Linda S. 1997. 'Why g matters: The complexity of everyday life', in *Intelligence*, 24 (1): 79-132.

Caspi, Avshalom. 2002. 'Role of genotype in the cycle of violence in maltreated children', in *Science*, 297: 851-854.

Coates, John M. and Joe Herbert. 2008. 'Endogenous steroids and financial risk taking on a London trading floor', in *Proceedings of the National Academy of Sciences*, 105: 6167-6172.

DSM-III-R. 1987. *Diagnostic and Statistical Manual of Mental Disorders*. Arlington: VA: The American Psychiatric Association.

Fukuyama, Francis. 2004. 'Transhumanism', in *Foreign Policy* (September-October 2004). Available at http://www.foreignpolicy.com/articles/2004/09/01/transhumanism. Accessed November 27 2011.

Gottfredson, Linda S. 1997. 'Why g matters: The complexity of everyday life', in *Intelligence*, 24(1): 79-132. Viewed July 3rd 2009. http://www.udel.edu/educ/gottfredson/reprints/1997whygmatters.pdf.

Lim, M. M. et al. 2004. 'Enhanced partner preference in a promiscuous species by manipulating the expression of a single gene', in *Nature* 429: 754-757.

Mackie, John. 1984. 'Rights, Utility, and Universalization' in *Utility and Right*, ed. R.G. Frey. Minneapolis: University of Minnesota Press.

Maher, B. 2008. 'Poll results: Look who's doping', in *Nature* 452: 674-675.

Mischel, Walter et al. 1988. 'The nature of adolescent competencies predicted by preschool delay of gratification', in *Journal of Personality & Social Psychology* 54 (4): 687-696.

Narcissistic Personality Disorder Forum. 2011. Accessed 13 January 2011 at http://forum2.aimoo.com/NARCISSISTICPERSONALITYDISORDER/m/Targets-Speak-Out-Read-Only/High-Risk-Children-1-1035612.html.

Parfit, Derek. 1997. 'Equality or Priority?', in *Ratio* vol. 10, Issue 3: 202-221.

Rawls, John A. 1971. *Theory of Justice*. Cambridge: Harvard University Press.

Sandel, Michael. 2004. 'The Case Against Perfection', in *Atlantic Monthly*. April 2004: 51-62.

Savulescu, J. (1994). 'Rational Desires and the Limitation of Life-Sustaining Treatment', in *Bioethics* 8: 191-222.

Savulescu, Julian. 1995. 'Rational Non-Interventional Paternalism: Why Doctors Ought to Make Judgements of What Is Best for Their Patients', in *Journal of Medical Ethics* 21: 327-331.

Savulescu, Julian. 1997. 'Liberal Rationalism and Medical Decision-Making', in *Bioethics* 11: 115-129.

Savulescu, Julian. 2001. 'Procreative Beneficence: Why We Should Select the Best Children', in *Bioethics*
vol.15 (5): 413-426.

Savulescu, Julian. 2006. 'Genetic Interventions and the Ethics of Enhancement of Human Beings', in
The Oxford Handbook of Bioethics, ed. Bonnie Steinbock, 516-535. Oxford: Oxford University Press.

Savulescu, Julian. 2007. 'Autonomy, the Good Life, and Controversial Choices', in *The Blackwell Guide
to Medical Ethics*, eds. Rosamond Rhodes et al. Oxford: Blackwell Publishing.

Savulescu, Julian. 2009. 'Enhancement and Fairness', in *Unnatural Selection: The Challenges of Engineering
Tomorrow's People*, eds. Healey, Peter and Steve Rayner. London: Earthscan.

Savulescu, Julian. 2009. 'Genetic Enhancement', in *A Companion to Bioethics*, eds. Helga Kuhse and
Peter Singer. Oxford: Blackwell Publishing.

Savulescu, Julian. 2010. 'Human liberation: Removing biological and psychological barriers to freedom',
in *Monash Bioethics Review* vol. 29 (1).

Savulescu, Julian and Guy Kahane. 2009. 'The Moral Obligation to Create Children with the Best Chance
of the Best Life', in *Bioethics* vol. 23 (5): 274-290.

Savulescu, Julian and Richard W. Momeyer. 1997. 'Should Informed Consent Be Based on Rational
Beliefs?', in *Journal of Medical Ethics* 23 (5): 282-288.

Savulescu, Julian and Anders Sandberg. 2007. 'The Neuroenhancement of Love and Marriage: The
Chemicals Between Us', in *Neuroethics*, 1: 31-44.

Singer, P. 1985. 'All Animals Are Equal', in *Applied Ethics*, ed. Peter Singer. Oxford: Oxford University Press.

Walum, Hasse et al. 2008. 'Genetic Variations in the Vasopressin Receptor 1a Gene (AVPR1A) Associ-
ates with Pair Bonding Behaviour in Humans', in *Proceedings of the National Academy of Science*
105 (37): 14153-14156.

Winslow, J.T. et al. 1993. 'A role for central vasopressin in pair bonding in monogamous prairie voles',
in *Nature* 365: 545-548.

Young, L.J. et al. 1999. 'Increased affiliative response to vasopressin in mice expressing the V1a receptor
from a monogamous vole', in *Nature* 400: 766-768.

Index

I

identity   10, 12, 14, 16, 50, 58, 82-
    86, 111, 120, 123-124, 129, 147
ideology   54, 150, 161, 190
illegality   15, 93, 180
illnesses, see diseases
illusions   35, 125
IMAGEN   49
imagination   33-34, 117-118, 124,
    127, 136, 139
immigration   160
immortality   13-14, 20, 29, 39-40,
    69, 76, 82, 98, 125
immune system   27, 40, 42, 63
impermissibility   15, 93, 96-97, 101,
    109
implanted devices   68
impulse control   188, 198
in-group   195-196
inanimate natural objects   161-162
incremental improvements   117
individualists   56
individuality   134
industrialization   38, 129, 157
inequality   65-66, 70-71, 106, 162,
    182, 184-186, 188, 192-193,
    196-197, 199, 201
inevitability   29, 155, 157
infant-parent relationship   199
inferior frontal cortex   194
inferior parietal lobule   194
information society   128, 139
inheritance   33, 58
injuries   65, 68, 177
injustice   90, 98
innovation   19-20, 28, 31, 57, 65-66,
    128, 158, 160, 165-166, 168
inorganic matter   118
insects   27
instrument mechanics   130

insula neurons   194
insulin   63
intellectual
    disability   188
    diversity   56
intelligence   11, 26, 39, 45, 55, 112-
    113, 118, 130, 161-163, 170,
    172-176, 178, 180-182, 184,
    188-189, 201
    gaps   55
    general 188
    low   178, 180-181, 189
    tests   178
interactive experiments   16
interiorization   148
internal cognitive enhancements   68
International Classification of Disease
    (ICD)   65
international regulation   118, 167-168
internationalization   167
internet   16, 27, 35, 68, 137-138,
    152, 168, 190
interpretation   53, 84
intersections   75, 190
intersex condition   197
interweb   33, 35
intolerance   8, 100
Inuits   54
inviolable core characteristics   83
iodine 190
IQ   17, 55, 170, 173, 175-177, 188-
    193
Ishiguro, Kazuo   125-126

J

Jamison, Andrew   26, 34
Jehova's Witnesses   111
Jesuits   149
Jordan, Michael   182
Judaeo-Christian doctrines   166